The ONE Diet

Georges Philips & Simon Shawcross

Published by Copeland and Wickson

The ONE Diet

First published 2011

ISBN-13: 978-1904928010
ISBN-10: 1904928013

www.theonediet.com

Before commencing this or any diet and/or exercise program, discuss the matter with your medical doctor to ensure that there are no medical concerns that make dieting or exercise unsuitable. The contents of this book are for educational purposes only and are not intended as medical advice. The publishers, editors, and authors cannot accept any responsibility for consequences arising from the use of information contained within this book.

Dedicated to my grandparents Allen and Edna Wickson

Simon Shawcross

Foreword

The ONE Diet is a perfect name for the book you are about to read. It is not just another in a long string of diets that you have tried…it is THE diet that correlates with the genome within your body that has been evolving over billions of years.

Go get a new roll of toilet paper. Look at it. Let this entire roll represent the history of the human species. Holding the roll in your left hand, tear off a single square of the tissue and hold it in your right hand. What you hold in your left hand represents the amount of time that our species lived off the land as hunter-gatherers. What you hold in your right hand represents the agricultural revolution.

Now, take the square that you hold in your right hand and use a razor blade to cut off the tiniest sliver from the end that you can manage. This tiny sliver represents the twentieth and twenty-first centuries. This is the slice of time where you will live out your life. Within this slice is a growing epidemic of obesity, diabetes, hypertension, heart disease, and depression. Also within this slice is every diet book that has tried to address this problem, using various manipulations of foodstuffs from the agricultural revolution.

Now let us return to the roll of tissue that you are holding in your left hand. Over this entire span of time, there was not a single obese human. Humans like every other animal, autoregulated to an ideal body composition without even thinking about it. Along with the lack of obesity, anthropologic evidence suggests that the diseases that track along with obesity (diabetes, hypertension, heart disease, etc.) were also not present. Throughout this expanse of time free of obesity and disease, there was just ONE diet. The ONE diet was a hunter-gatherer diet.

The ONE Diet will take you on a journey that begins at the ending. In order to make room in your mind for what the diet that shaped your genome looks like, the authors first must do some house cleaning. My dear friend and co-author John Little is also the authorized biographer of Bruce Lee. I remember watching a video interview of Bruce Lee with John when he was discussing how best to teach a pupil. He likened the learning process to a tea ceremony. Both participants in the tea ceremony have tea in their cups. In order for a teacher to give a pupil his tea, the pupil must be willing to pour his tea out of his cup.

Mr. Philips and Mr. Shawcross also realize the importance of this concept and will painstakingly show you what is wrong with the contemporary Western diet and how it foils your attempts to achieve a healthy body composition. They will show you how and why you have been frustrated. More importantly, they will show how your frustration has been used by marketers and scam artists to manipulate you and get your money.

Having dispelled the "conventional wisdom" that has grown out of the experience within that tiny sliver of time in your right hand, *The ONE Diet* will end at the beginning. The authors will explain what the diet that drove the development of your genome looked like. Once they show you what that diet looked like, they will show how to approximate it in the modern environment. Rather than simply suggesting "Paleo re-enactment," the authors will show you what to avoid in the modern environment and what to include so that the correct metabolic and hormonal environment exists.

One of my favorite aspects of this book is that it focuses on an aspect of body recomposition that all the other books in the Paleo genre have largely ignored: the psychological aspect. The authors understand that no matter how powerful the arguments, or how deep your understanding, if you have unresolved psychological issues you are doomed to failure. Throughout *The ONE Diet*, there are discussions of the potential psychological roadblocks and strategies for how to overcome them.

One of my major dissatisfactions with other books advocating an evolutionary-based diet is that after giving a beautiful treatise shattering the conventional wisdom on diet, they would launch into a discussion of exercise that involved a conventional wisdom that was as inaccurate as the diet they just debunked. Not so with *The ONE Diet*. The authors correctly recommend a high intensity program that is brief and infrequent. Such an approach to exercise creates an optimal metabolic and hormonal environment that will work synergistically with your new diet without creating overtraining or burnout. And rather than trying to cover the exercise topic as extensively as the diet, they simply outline a solid starting point and make appropriate references for readers who want more.

You now hold in your hands *The ONE Diet*. It is NOT the next new thing. It is a very old thing…billions of years in the making. It is what drove the evolution of the genome which makes up your body. It cannot fail. As the philosopher, Francis Bacon said: "Nature, to be commanded, must be obeyed."

In Health and Strength,

M. Doug McGuff, MD
Co-Author of *Body by Science*

Chapter 1.
The Miracle Industry

IN A NUTSHELL:

- There are many gimmicky products, books, and services out there looking to capture a portion of the weight loss market. Be aware that you don't fall prey to their outlandish claims. The weight loss industry is now worth between $33 billion and $55 billion per year in the United States alone.

- In the West, we are often held to ransom between a food industry that continually supplies an overabundance of the wrong foods and a miracle weight loss industry promising to solve our weight issues "overnight." No product or service can better a natural, healthy diet that you adhere to over the long term.

- Models used in advertising to promote unhealthy foods are never overweight; they always appear slim, happy, and smiling. Modeling is a profession; they are paid well to remain in good shape, stay lean, and smile.

- Almost any diet approach may appear effective in the first four weeks or so due to the body's release of excess water and recovery from systemic inflammation.

- Water loss can account for two to ten pounds per week of weight lost in the first few weeks of a diet, and many popular diets rely on this to appear effective.

- If you are truly prepared to do what is required to healthily lose weight and keep it off, all the information you need is contained within *The ONE Diet*.

Cʒ

"For all their virtues, markets often give companies a strong incentive to cater to (and profit from) human frailties, rather than to try to eradicate them or to minimize their effects."

Richard H. Thaler and Cass R. Sunstein, *Nudge*

Every year Americans spend between $33 billion and $55 billion on all manner of weight loss products and services. The trend is similar throughout the rest of the Western world. A multitude of apparent options vie for the attention of the prospective consumer, from "special" berries and teas, fad diets, exercise regimens, medical procedures, pills, and potions, to weight loss groups and e-books.

We suggest that the majority of those products and services will not get you to where you want to be, and most of that money is unfortunately, poured down the drain. The real winner of the weight loss world is usually the weight loss industry itself, not the individuals who fund it with their desire to become thinner, slim, or healthy.

The super-fast-paced world in which we now live, with its proliferation of fast-grown, fast-raised, fast-packed, low-nutrient fast food fosters a desire for instant, easy solutions that don't require us to change our lifestyles or comfort eating patterns.

The promise that a pill, a gadget, or some recently discovered and overpriced exotic berry will change us from fat to thin overnight is the bait the weight loss industry knows will ensnare its often unaware and sometimes desperate target audience.

Apparent "scientific studies" are occasionally presented to "prove" the weight loss efficacy of some newly found or synthesized substance. Yet those who actually read the small print rather than believe the oh-so-appealing hype will see that the difference between eating a well-rounded and healthy diet and spending hundreds of dollars or pounds on the new gimmick pill is infinitesimally small. That, of course, is if we even believe the research (often funded by the company that manufactures the product) is valid in the first place...

Of course, in those studies, the subjects using the super kaka berry, or whatever is being sold, did eat a very well-controlled diet. Unlike those who buy the product and often continue to eat the same way they always have, innocently believing the advertising hype and questionable before-and-after images. When the product has failed for them, they'll have to notch it down to experience, often blaming themselves rather than the product.

We want to save you from all that disappointment and hassle. Know that if you want sustainable and healthy weight loss, there is no superconvenient short cut. It is likely you will have to change the way you eat somewhat and alter your lifestyle to a degree.

Even people who undergo extreme operations, like gastric banding, can get around having a smaller available stomach size. They often adapt by consuming more sugary foods and liquids, such as sodas, fruit juices, and rich desserts. Individuals who have gastric bands fitted can often surpass the initial discomfort of eating too much for their stomachs' reduced capacities, anyway.

Pills, kaka berries and electrical belts are unlikely to lead you down the valued path of sustainable weight loss. If the gimmick method is the route a person is persuaded to take, he or she had best be prepared to make friends with his or her fat, because it will probably be around for a lifetime.

It is easy to think that we can just change, that it's easy to achieve our desired weight with a "miracle" plan or product. Just pop a few pills, rub some cream on, eat some more fruit from the magical forest, and all the fat will simply go away. And pigs may fly.

human body has evolved to eat, as outlined in *The ONE Diet*.

If you really want to lose your body fat, you can rest your mind, stop the search, put a stake in the ground, and finally say enough is enough.

You can firmly say no to any more pills, stimulants, diuretics, powders, shakes, soups and very low-calorie diets. You can walk away from the latest slew of unproven, but "scientific" sounding and trendy diets claiming to be the next new thing that doubtless would leave you disappointed after a few weeks anyway.

You won't need to buy weird berries or "special" oriental teas, and you won't have to be misled by food-industry-funded, government recommendations. We want to help save your money and time from being wasted: on electrical belts, vibrating machines, hours of "aerobic" exercise, or whatever other gimmicks are thrown at you, repackaged, or invented to sell you in the future. No matter what star does it, athlete recommends it, or PhD puts his or her name to it.

Stop, breathe, relax, clear your mind, smile, and know that you've found a healthy, sustainable and natural approach to weight loss now…the search is over.

If you really want to lose your excess weight, all the information you need is now at your fingertips. The question is, is the cost worth it to you, the cost of changing your old nutritional habits as best you can? Well, that is a question only you can answer. If your answer is yes, then read on…

ଔ

IN CONCLUSION:

- Stay focused and alert to the various methods used to bring to your attention "miracle cures."

- In the old days, "miracle snake oil" salesmen were chased out of town or worse. Regrettably, that is no longer legal. The best we can do is not give any of our precious attention to such hogwash.

- Stay as pure to your needs as your purse allows. Through your actions, you can teach your world that you are not prepared to accept kaka foods, nor will you support the growth of an industry that puts profit before people.

- Very low-calorie diets are often a problematic approach to weight loss.

- The ONE Diet will enable you to achieve your ideal weight naturally.

addicted to are extremely dangerous to the longevity and quality of our lives.

Addictions to most feel-good substances have long been known and accepted as being dangerous. We are so susceptible to things that bring about instant gratification that it does not take much thinking to understand how easy it is for some to be addicted to fast-acting street and prescription drugs.

Addictions, which include dependencies such as cocaine and heroin, are well known to affect some people more than others. One person can smoke an illegal substance now and then, a sort of take-it-or-leave-it attitude, whilst another, once started, will find it difficult to stop without help from a professional.

We joke about people being chocoholics and alcoholics. It seems to have become social and acceptable to engage in amounts that common sense tells us is dangerous. Often it is only when we are told by an expert that we are going to die that we take it seriously enough to do something about it. The shock of termination can have that effect.

How Your Weekly Food Budget is Targeted

Modern food companies have teams of researchers and marketers whose job it is to find ways of selling us something at a profit. The more they can get us hooked on their product, the better the investment return. We may then, be classed as loyal customers or, from another perspective, addicts.

Brand loyalty is an area where vast sums of money are spent, to ensure that we remain loyal (addicted) to their brand. Generations have grown up buying things because their parents bought them, due to clever advertising they were exposed to years ago.

It can even appear that your loyalty will be rewarded with extra points and bonuses. This "buy-in" is very sophisticated and appears to be innocent, whilst in reality, information is collected so as to observe buying habits and predict future areas of sales. But hey, we are getting those triple points and think we are getting something for free; in fact, we are allowing the hook to sink deeply into our gullets.

Placement advertising occurs when corporations pay filmmakers and others to ensure that they place their products so that the viewer has sight of them in a subtle setting. It is a covert, if not a subversive method of duping us into believing that people prefer to use a particular product, and our minds accept this as social proof. The consequences are that we are likely to view this as the norm and more readily buy into the product sold to us.

Getting rid of excess fat is about untangling the myths and misconceptions that have been so carefully planted into our psyches in such a way that we have become incapable of recognizing the truth even if it lands at our feet.

This book goes some way to help get things into context if we are ever to get control of our bodies. The important thing is to make informed decisions on what, if any, your addictions may be and to understand the cost to your life.

An old business adage goes something like this: if you know what someone wants and you can sell it to him or her at a profit, then what are you waiting for? That is all that happens. When an opportunity arises, corporations will take advantage. It is the way of the world; it's not personal, it's just business. The larger the profit, the more successful the business, the more sustainable, and the longer it will survive.

Losing fat weight is our end goal. For some of us this will be challenging. We are facing a difficult time ahead. By regaining the power to buy and cook real food, we will have engaged in a personal empowerment revolution.

What we know is that our minds are very easily programmable. This is not, however, something that we want to believe about ourselves. Nonetheless, it is *a fact of life*. The degree of programmability, though variable from one person to another, nevertheless exists for all and is inescapable, particularly through our formative years.

It is this knowledge that advertisers use to control our purchasing power. We are individuals with perceived powers of choice, yet we rarely analyze our choices. We develop relationships with just about everything in our lives.

A brand leader is a brand leader because it has succeeded in finding or creating a niche in our common minds and has filled it with a desire that it then goes on to provide. The advertisers have learnt our buttons and know which to press and which to avoid.

Once we have been switched on to an idea and that idea has taken root in our minds, it becomes interwoven in our psyche in such a way that we often cannot discriminate between thoughts that are self-deduced and those implanted by another. It just becomes part of us.

Once the idea "best burger in the universe" has been established in our minds, it becomes protected by our own mind's mechanism. It has a wonderful way of maintaining its truths. There are processes that make it possible for the mind to keep truths stable and consistent.

Food has become a major feature in our everyday life. We seem to be surrounded by it; on billboards, magazines, Internet, television, radio, and so on. It seems that we are swimming in it. Endless streets of food retail outlets; hot-dog vendors, burger bars, chicken shacks, Chinese, Mexican, Indian restaurants, etc.

Our ability to be influenced is a pivotal part of our existence, and one that is not sufficiently explored through education. The tendency is to believe that we decide what to think, and that when someone tells us something, we can make our own decisions.

In some cases, when we are aware of what is happening, we will use our mental process to think and weigh up the benefits of what is being proposed, evaluate, and conclude. It is, however, extremely difficult to be constantly aware of external influences.

Keeping up a shield takes energy that could eventually cause exhaustion. We are often beaten by the sheer volume of advertising that is coming at us from all directions, designed to get to our senses with pinpoint accuracy and precision. Only the well informed and willful seem to be able to reject this onslaught and defend their minds and bodies.

The tendency is to go with the flow and fit in with whatever is going on around us. It saves us having to work things out if someone else has done it for us. Our desire to fit in often precludes us doing what is right and good. The thing is, what's popular is not necessarily what's good, and what's good is not always popular.

Consider the fashion industry and how it governs many people's lives. The trendsetters often dictate what most of us end up wearing. The style, color, length, and the brand logo are just some of the things that we are influenced by. The irony is that once we decide to fit in, we are hostage to the system that we have chosen to fit in to.

This all starts very early on in our lives. Consider the times at kindergarten when one child sees another holding a toy and then tells a parent that he or she, too, wants one. Children see an elder child refuse to eat carrots, and the next thing you know they do not like carrots. It doesn't look cool eating what others reject.

Often we can see how children react when they are introduced to a brand of burger which has a little toy collection or similar prize given away every time they have the "meal." It's not that they want the meal, but rather that they want the toy. It doesn't take long to get them to desire the fast-fattening food.

Advertising Works!

Why do the advertised images look so much better than the real thing? To entice us into tasting our imagination and desiring what we sight-tasted. Perhaps our imagination was hijacked into thinking that we were going to eat what we saw. Advertising really does work.

"Can you imagine a lemon? It is perfectly yellow. Imagine it in your hands and just sense the texture of the skin. Imagine bringing it to your nose and smelling its scent. Now imagine you will cut it in half, and just observe the juice dripping slightly. Imagine that you will taste the juice and perhaps even cut a slice and taste it. As you bite into it and you sink your teeth into the segment, the sharp flavor erupts into your mouth."

As you read the above paragraph, you may have noticed that you were likely to have begun to salivate. Yet there was no lemon in reality. That is the power of the imagination once it is stimulated into action. Keep in mind that when corporations are aiming their products at us, we are likely to be seduced by the advertising. It is just the nature of things; it's not personal, it's just business.

Subliminal information is infecting us most of the time. Perhaps we may understand it better by exploring why so many corporations and the like spend vast amounts of money on advertising. It is not because they want to keep the magazines in business, nor their preferred Internet browser alive, nor is it that they want you to be entertained by the latest design out of their creative department.

Advertisers are there to grab our attention. Our attention is worth a fortune, and the company depends on getting our attention. There is a whole raft of graduates paid to come up with ways to capture our attention, people such as creative directors, marketers, and other specialists in mind control.

You may think "Yeah, and?" The "Yeah, and?" is that once they have our attention, they have created a window of opportunity. If they can create a large enough window in our minds, they can climb in and start setting out their store.

There is little that we have not been programmed to accept as being our opinion. There is a very divisive strategy in operation. Let us convince you that you are making the right choice when you buy our product. They can rest at ease once we have made a connection with the brand, especially when we start promoting it to our friends. Loyalty is the "cherry on the cake" for most organizations.

We can also be played with, when it comes to statistics. There are so many corporations that use statistics to convince our weaned mind. When we hear that 68 percent of the people preferred a particular product to any other brand, we may dismiss the statistic consciously, yet a remnant often remains at the subconscious level.

We need to take a moment and consider the freebies that we are offered at the supermarket. Taste this, use our free offer, start collecting these tokens and every time you get ten you can get one free.

Occasionally it would be prudent to remind ourselves that these companies' objective is to run their companies at a profit. Without profit there is no company. It is not about our survival, it is about their prosperity. It can all start to feel like these companies really care about us, and we then, on some level, stop being aware of what is being sold to us. We have slowly dropped our guard and just accepted that this is acceptable. Any angle that can be used to manipulate our thinking and control our choices will be used.

We are living in a no-holds-barred world where market forces are competing for our income. It is without doubt about profit. Now the question needs to be: what can we do about this, as individuals who want to design a healthy lifestyle?

We are trapped by our own tendency to get away with doing the least possible. "Let's get little tables so that we can sit in front of the television and eat dinner (whilst being sold more things)." We might say to those who challenge our behavior that we are more sophisticated than that and we are not affected by the adverts.

Unfortunately, we have all been well and truly had. *Our minds have a limited antivirus system. Once our subconscious mind has been breached, our mental firewall is ineffective.*

Most people are trapped in a vicious cycle of eating what is in front of them with little thought beyond the immediate taste. There is a difference between a food that tastes good, and a food that tastes good *and* does us good.

If you met a person who wears a perfume that smells nice to you, would that make her a nice person? If a dealer is giving you an extra year's road cover on a new car, would that make it a safer car, a better car?

Good Companies *Are* Out There

The fight for real food is almost over. There are just a few glimmers of hope left here and there, and we applaud those who look to make a profit by providing something that is actually healthy for us at a sensible price.

Forward-thinking food producers are few, and we need to celebrate them wherever and whenever we can. In this day and age, they tend to be struggling to compete with the conglomerates. It is not going to be easy to survive the fast-food revolution, if it can be survived at all. The thought that our children and those to come after will be enslaved into addiction is scary.

To maintain a healthier body and consequently a calmer mind, we will be required to be vigilant and deliberate in our efforts to control substances that enter our diet which overly stimulate and damage our bodies.

The art is to develop an attitude and state of mind that challenges all that is being offered to us. It is prudent to ask, "What's in it for them?" Challenge absolutely everything.

If we spent as much time thinking about and shopping for healthy foods as we do thinking about what bath oils we are going to use, what makeup, what lipstick, what scent, what clothing, etc., we might find that we make a massive improvement in our general well-being.

We are lost in brands and motifs and often live by the next craze that hits the streets. Everything from fliers to personalized e-mails bombards not only our clothing habits, but also our eating habits. It is as if we have become sitting targets for marketers who want to have their way with us, without consideration or any responsibilities for the consequences.

Slurp drinks made of sweet gunk have become the standard. Supersize this, supersize that, and continue until we are all supersized. The trick, if you are in the business of selling food, is to provide the customer with that magical ingredient that keeps them coming back for more.

We might confuse the suppliers/manufacturers of mass-market foods as legal dealers and that we are trained to perform on their advertising call. It is concerning how easily influenced we are. We are scared at the thought of not fitting in with those around us and scared of not being seen as individuals.

We need to retrieve the responsibility and get back to the reality that if we stop caring, we are in danger of not having any control over what happens to us.

ଔ

IN CONCLUSION:

- No person, organization, corporation, or government can be relied on to have our best interests at heart. It is up to us to champion our self-interest and challenge all information presented to us.

- Conflicting messages and the use of disinformation and corporate spin have infiltrated and infected our notion of eating well.

- By having the right information, we can make better choices and avoid being stuck in a web of deception. Consuming real food and avoiding processed products will improve the quality of our life and make our weight loss goals obtainable.

- Challenging our own beliefs, our habitual shopping behavior, as well the information presented to us is now vital if we are to be free of the illusions.

Chapter 3.
What's Really Going Wrong

IN A NUTSHELL:

- The problem of obesity and weight gain in today's world lies in the dramatic increase in the consumption of calories derived from refined carbohydrates (primarily from grains, sugars, and sweeteners).

- Modern chemically altered sweeteners, like high fructose corn syrup, that are major ingredients in many processed foods and drinks substantially compound this problem.

- The vast majority of the food industry focuses on maximizing profit by selling us cheap-to-produce "foods" and "drinks" loaded with refined carbohydrates. These processed foods are far removed from being "real foods."

- Low-quality and processed foods can stimulate increased hunger and, in some cases, may send us into an eating frenzy. Refined carbohydrates for instance can have similar physiological, addictive effects to recreational drugs.

ଔ

"Historically, we never consumed much sugar. We're not built to process it."

Barry Popkin, Professor of Nutrition at the University of North Carolina

In our modern era, we need to ask ourselves: what is causing the excess weight gain epidemic that is negatively affecting so many of us? The straightforward answer to that question is refined carbohydrates, grains, and added sugars. These are foods or ingredients that our human species originally didn't eat at all, or could not eat in any great quantity because of their rarity in the natural environment.

It was not until the commencement of the first agricultural revolution about ten thousand years ago that consumption of grains and refined sugars began to become widespread in the human diet. Although ten thousand years may initially seem a long period of time to some readers, it is a drop in the ocean in terms of human evolution.

What Are Carbohydrates?

Simply put, carbohydrates are sugars and starches (starches are the more complex sugars).

The Major Sources of Rapidly Digested Carbohydrates in the Modern World:

GRAINS—Cereal grains, whole grains, refined grains, flours, and products that are made from or contain grains (pasta, bread, breakfast cereals, pastries, biscuits, crackers, pies and other bakery goods, etc.).

SUGARS AND SWEETENERS—Foods and drinks that contain added sugars and sweeteners: sugar, sucrose, dextrose, fructose, high fructose corn syrup, rice syrup, glucose, and so on. (These sweeteners are present in ready meals, cakes, biscuits, jams, confectionary, desserts, sodas, soft drinks, sports/energy drinks, etc.).

JUNK FOOD IN GENERAL—Ready meals, microwave meals, crisps, chocolate, crackers, fast food/junk food, soft drinks, etc. Some of these "foods" contain grains *and* sugars/sweeteners!

Consider that for around 150,000 generations of human existence, refined and junk foods were not within constant reach the moment people felt pangs of hunger. In addition, it is only in the last three or four generations, in the West in particular, that an overabundance of processed high-carbohydrate snacks and drinks has been proliferated.

Our bodies have not evolved to be able to cope with this much and this type of food. Many of us end up feeling guilty for overeating or eating an excess of the wrong types of food. This guilt is then compounded by the expectations of what we feel we ought to look like, as presented by images in the media.

The vast majority of the food we in the West, consume today is based on or contains large amounts of refined grains, refined carbohydrates, and sugars. Many of us end up fat, often turning to "miracle" diets/products, drugs, or surgical procedures in an attempt to regain our natural shape. This is akin to putting a plaster over a wound we ourselves are continually and often unknowingly aggravating by consuming the "foods" of modern commerce.

Sugar Intake is Still Increasing

Sugar intake alone in the Western world has certainly spiraled out of control. Research carried out by the Center for Science in the Public Interest has shown that Americans today consume 28 percent more sugar than just a few decades ago in 1983.[1] That is a massive increase for such a short period. Further statistics from the U.S. Department of Agriculture highlight that the typical American eats 20 teaspoons of added sugar every day (this figure does not include fructose or lactose that naturally occurs in fruit and milk). That's around 100 grams (or 400 calories) of added, unhealthy, nutritionally empty, simple sugar carbohydrates a day. No wonder there is an ongoing epidemic of obesity.

Weight Gain: Driven by the Modern Diet

We believe that many of society's advancements are fantastic. We are continually saving labor and improving the dissemination of information; our understanding of the world around us is getting better in many respects, and Western medicine, in terms of emergency interventions, is simply awesome.

However, in the fields of food production, food manufacture, food advertising, and Western medicine's attempts to treat chronic diseases caused by the modern diet, we are failing big time.

According to recent research on our nutritional history, throughout approximately 99.6 percent of our species' evolutionary development from some three million years ago until about ten thousand years ago, our forebears' diet consisted of "meats, seafood, fresh fruits, and fresh vegetables."[2] It is these foods that can truly be considered the original, natural, health-giving human diet.

The reason we have a greater problem with obesity in today's world is not primarily due to a lack of exercise. It is the sheer overabundance of food, especially nutritionally empty, processed food, which is causing many of us to gain excess weight.

We have become unwitting victims of industrialized agriculture and food manufacturers whose mission statement may be "Maximize cheap fillers, maximize profit margin, and minimize nutritional value, because people are too confused or not aware of what we put in our products nowadays, nor of the effect it has on their bodies anymore."

We are not against the producers and manufacturers of industrialized agriculture and food production. They are extremely effective at what they do: providing cheap food for a massive market. They run their businesses from a money-making and profit- maximizing point of view, and do so extremely well, and they market their products with great sophistication.

Refined carbohydrates are the cheapest ingredients on the modern menu, and they are everywhere in plenty—soft drinks, fruit juices, pasta, bread, and hidden away in ready meals and snacks. According to Larry Johnson, a food scientist at the University of Iowa Center for Crops Utilization, about 90 percent of food on the typical supermarket shelf "would contain either a corn or a soybean ingredient, and most of the time it will contain both."[3]

Perhaps we can now get the best of both worlds—the safety and protection of our modern environments, relatively low wear and tear on our bodies, the fallback of modern emergency medicine should we become injured, *and* the healthy way of eating that our ancestors enjoyed. We truly would be using our most evolutionarily important tool, our brain, if we are smart enough to do that.

As an individual, you have a choice to make: do you want to consume what has become the norm, what has become accepted as our daily food? Or do you want to consume life-giving natural foods that your body was designed to thrive on? Perhaps the human race will not always have this luxury of choice, but whilst we do have a choice, maybe it is wise to consider our options and choose what is best for us.

Grains and sugars are the ultimate cheap fillers that increase our likelihood of gaining fat and put us at greater risk of developing diabetes and the other conditions of metabolic syndrome.

What is Metabolic Syndrome/Syndrome X?

Simply put metabolic syndrome, or syndrome X, are the names given to a collection of interrelated diseases, conditions, and health issues caused primarily by the modern diet. Recent research also suggests that some people may have a genetic predisposition to developing metabolic syndrome, which makes eating the right foods even more pertinent.[4]

The collection of health issues that make up the metabolic syndrome include obesity, cardiovascular disease, hypertension, diabetes, stroke, cancers, peptic ulcers, appendicitis, periodontal disease, gallstones, diverticulitis, varicose veins, hemorrhoids, constipation, and tooth cavities.

Studies of the remains of preagricultural man and observational studies of the few remaining hunter-gatherer tribes suggest that these diseases do not occur to any notable extent in humans until the introduction of refined sugars and grains as major components of our diet.[5]

These issues have been compounded in more recent times by the proliferation of junk foods and the addition of plant/vegetable oils, hydrogenated fats, and chemically altered sweeteners such as high fructose corn syrup (more to come on these later).

If You Want to Get Fat, Eat Like a Sumo Wrestler

It is interesting to note that in instances where deliberate excess weight gain is a goal, such as with the Massa tribe during the male fattening ritual and in Japanese sumo wrestlers, it is sugars and starches that are emphasized to excess in the diet, to elicit fat gain.

For the Massa, this comes in the form of milk and sorghum porridge (made from a relative of the sugar cane plant). And the sumo's diet typically consists of 57 percent–80 percent carbohydrates, primarily from large amounts of rice (often five bowls at each meal), by the way, typically only 9 percent–16 percent of their diets are made up of fat.

How the Food We Eat is Stored as Energy

Insulin

The hormone insulin is vital to the functioning of our body, as it is the major nutrient storage hormone. Insulin's main role is to process or store away blood sugar (also known as glucose), which has been derived from the food we consume. Too much glucose in our blood has a negative, toxic effect on the body.

Insulin's role also goes beyond this, as it is a key regulator of our metabolism, of glycogen synthesis (glycogen is synthesized from glucose and stored in the body as a reserve form of energy), and of fat synthesis and storage.

How Insulin Works

Upon eating, insulin is released from the pancreas. Insulin then has the effect of reducing other nutrients in our blood, stimulating hunger, and preparing us for the arrival of new glucose energy.

Energy from the food we have consumed is absorbed into the bloodstream, raising our blood sugar levels; this, in turn, stimulates the pancreas to release even more insulin.[6]

Insulin is secreted at this point, as it is required to shift the glucose (the blood sugar) into the cells of the body for storage. Once this has occurred, the blood glucose level is now in balance again.

Glycogen

Glycogen is the limited supply of ready energy that the body can store for use for our immediate energy needs. If you were to *avoid* consuming any food for a period, your body could run off its stored glycogen for about twelve to fourteen hours so long as you are relatively sedentary during that time.

If you were to continue not eating, to the point where you had used up all your stored glycogen, it would actually take you around twenty-four hours from the time you begin eating again until your body processes that energy and refills its glycogen stores.

Most people, however, never use up all their glycogen stores. In fact, for many individuals, their glycogen stores are full all of the time. This has big implications for weight gain and weight loss, as we shall see.

The human body can only store a limited amount of glycogen. The amount of glycogen you can store is slightly variable depending on your age and sex. Typically, an adult can store about 70 grams of glycogen in the liver and another 250 grams in skeletal muscle.

If more glucose enters the blood when these stores are full, that energy has to go somewhere else. It is at this point that triacylglycerol (fat) is synthesized, ultimately meaning any excess glycogen will now be stored as body fat. This is how weight gain occurs.

The majority of excess calories that most people consume are derived from carbohydrates, particularly refined carbohydrates.

Practically speaking, eating over 150 grams or so of carbohydrates a day within the context of an otherwise balanced diet, is likely to lead to incremental weight gain for many people. Over 300 grams a day and we're usually looking at major continual weight gain. In the West, the tendency is to eat even more than that on a daily basis: up to and even beyond 500 grams per day for some people.

Even those who are not overweight need to be careful about the quantity of refined carbohydrates they consume. This is because although they may not be adding subcutaneous fat (the fat layer between the muscles and the skin), they can still be adding fat around the internal organs (visceral fat), which may lead to major health issues over the long term.

The example below demonstrates how a person may be consuming excessive amounts of carbohydrates in their daily diet:

Bowl of cereal with milk—50 g of carbohydrates

Double burger in a bun—41 g of carbohydrates

Medium french fries—42 g carbohydrates

Individual chocolate bar—43 g of carbohydrates

One liter of cola—109 g carbohydrates (there is the equivalent of 18 heaped teaspoons of table sugar in one liter of cola)

Margherita pizza—70 g carbohydrates

Total Carbohydrates—355 g

Even those who may think they are watching what they eat usually consume more than enough carbohydrates to cause weight gain:

Bowl of bran flakes with milk—40 g

Large glass of fruit juice—40 g

Plain bagel (no filling)—40 g

Chicken fajita "diet" wrap—40 g

Strawberry and banana smoothie—33 g

"Low-fat" chicken tikka masala ready meal—50 g

Naan bread—80 g

Total Carbohydrates—323 g

The processed and refined carbohydrates detailed in these examples represent low quality, nutritionally poor energy sources for the human metabolism which do not satisfy the body's nutritional needs. The knock-on effect is we eat more and still don't feel satisfied—this often encourages us to snack again, perhaps even soon after eating.

Due to this, many of us crave continual instant hits of food—it becomes very similar to physiological addiction. Sugar has been shown to have an almost identical effect to addictive recreational drugs in the way the brain responds to it.[7]

When we first start cutting the unhealthy refined carbohydrates out of our diet, some of us may feel short-term withdrawal symptoms—because we have literally been unknowing addicts of sugars.

Internal Starvation

A person who eats excess refined carbohydrates on a daily basis is literally making his or her body a more efficient fat storage machine.

When this happens, Doug McGuff, MD, explains, "You are now in the throes of the metabolic syndrome. Now your fat cells are a tissue colony with a competitive advantage. You now suffer from 'internal starvation.'"[8]

The concept of internal starvation is important to grasp, because in this scenario, no matter how much you eat, you don't feel that satisfied. This is because the body is not getting the nutrients it really needs from the low quality calories provided.

The food energy this person consumes is going primarily into fat storage, and for some individuals muscle mass and protein levels in the body are being lowered at the same time. This will cause a slowing of the metabolic rate, meaning it becomes even easier to add further excess weight.

In this scenario, the energy we need to live is taken directly from the food we eat, with the excess going into fat storage, so the body never gets the opportunity to use its own stored fat.

Those living this scenario will likely see their weight gradually and continually increase, and they will be feeling hungry most of the time, driving them to consume more. They are also far more likely to be attracted to refined carbohydrates and sweet foods. This is the perfect vicious cycle of fat gain, a key element of metabolic syndrome, or syndrome X.

Dr. McGuff elaborates that this sets up a chain of ongoing health problems beyond merely gaining weight: "It gets worse: Many of the circulating hormones your body relies on now will have glucose attached to them, and your body recognizes them as foreign and begins attacking them…and the glands that produce them (thyroid hormone being a prime example)."[9]

So Is It Possible to Eat Too Few Carbohydrates?

The carbohydrate intakes mentioned below are presented to give you an understanding of how differing amounts of carbohydrate affect weight gain and weight loss. Bear in mind that when you follow The ONE Diet, you won't have to count carbohydrates or calories; you will automatically be in the carbohydrate "sweet spot" for weight loss.

We know that for many people who have excess fat, eating over 150 grams of carbohydrates per day is likely to cause continued weight gain. We also know that eating fewer carbohydrates than that, ideally somewhere between 50 and 100 grams per day, will enable the majority of those people to reduce their fat to an optimal level consistently over time.

So what happens if a person eats even fewer than 50 grams of carbohydrates per day? With this little an amount of carbohydrate intake, the body has to synthesize an alternative fuel source for its ongoing energy needs. Ketones are then produced as a by-product when the body metabolizes fatty acids for energy in the liver and kidney.

Ketones and Ketosis Explained

Ketones cannot be stored for later use (whereas glucose and energy converted into fat can), so the ketones circulate in the bloodstream until they are used. Or, as is the case with any excess beyond that used for current energy requirements, they are excreted, largely through urine. When a person is at the point where he or she is naturally excreting ketones, that individual is in a state known as ketosis.

Being in ketosis is acceptable for a short period of time (twelve to forty-eight hours); it simply means that your body is running on converted protein rather than carbohydrates. Being in ketosis for periods longer than forty-eight hours is likely to put an unnecessary strain on the body, which is not something we would recommend as a healthy approach to weight loss for the majority of people. (There may be instances where a medically supervised ketosis diet is acceptable, such as for diabetics.)

Most people have no need to consume so few carbohydrates that ketosis is induced, to lose weight (which would effectively mean eliminating many healthy vegetables and fruits that contain relatively small amounts of naturally occurring sugars, in addition to eliminating the unhealthy grains and added sugars). Most people will lose weight plenty fast enough with a diet that includes vegetables and some fruit.

AN IN-DEPTH LOOK AT SOME OF THE KEY INGREDIENTS AND FOODS THAT ARE MAKING US FAT

Cereal Grains

"Generally, in most parts of the world, whenever cereal-based diets were first adopted as a staple food, replacing the primarily animal-based diets of hunter-gatherers, there was a characteristic reduction in stature, an increase in infant mortality, a reduction in lifespan, an increased incidence of infectious diseases, an increase in iron deficiency anemia, an increased incidence of...bone mineral disorders and an increase in the number of dental caries and enamel defects."

Loren Cordain[10]

In their natural state, grains, which are the seed head in plants such as wheat, are not digestible by humans. What agricultural man learned to do is to mill the grain, making it somewhat more digestible to us.

However, in doing this, the fibrous element of grain is largely removed—so when we consume flour (and products containing flour); we are eating a processed and refined source of carbohydrate that is of poor nutritional value.

As a side note, a similar occurrence happens with fruit juices, because the fiber has largely been removed from the fruit in the pressing/juicing process, what we are left with is an almost pure sugar drink.

Grains are really quite inedible; have you ever tried eating grains straight from the head of a wheat plant? As we have noted, for humans they need to be milled or ground and then cooked just to make them palatable and digestible by the human gastrointestinal (GI) tract.

A key issue with cereal grains is that they contain several antinutrients, including protease inhibitors, phytates, alkylresorcinols, and lectins. Lectins, for example have the effect of decreasing the intestinal absorption of many nutrients that are beneficial to us. In addition, what calcium there is in whole grain cereals is blocked from absorption by the phytates.

Wheat also contains gluten, which is a prolamine peptide and is indicated in many diseases now affecting the Western world, such as type 1 diabetes, celiac disease, multiple sclerosis, and rheumatoid arthritis.

When consumed in large amounts, as is typical in the modern Western diet, grains wreak havoc with most people's metabolism and health. As research scientist Loren Cordain notes, *"Many of the world's people suffer disease and dysfunction directly attributable to the consumption of these foods."*[11]

Our society has seen a large increase in calories consumed, notably since the 1970s, and these calories have largely come from carbohydrates derived from grains and sugar. The prevalence of grains and sugars in the typical Western diet is unprecedented in our history and is one of the major causes of excess fat, obesity, diabetes, and many more health ailments that affect our population.

A Further Note about Wheat Products

An article in the *Journal of Nutrition and Health* posits that modern wheat containing a low amount of selenium can depress the activity of the enzyme diodinase, which plays a vital part in the production of thyroid hormone. This makes cutting out wheat potentially important for those with thyroid issues.[12]

Wheat is Just Bad News

White flour and products made from white flour are plain and simply bad news for the human metabolism. White flour has had most of its nutrients processed out of it, leaving nothing but refined carbohydrates. Whole grain and whole grain products are still no better for us due to their greater antinutrient content, which stimulates intestinal distress and, over the longer term, can cause mineral deficiencies and other health issues.

So Why Do the Food Industry and Our Governments Promote Grains as Healthy Foods?

You may well be asking why our governments heavily promote the consumption of grains. Grains are typically a cheap crop to produce, with many influential vested interests involved in the business of grains all the way from seed bank to supermarket.

As a crop type, all cereals account annually for about 2,300 million metric tons (mmt) of food production—that is more than double the next most harvested crop type. What about the world's most produced individual crops? Sugar cane comes first at 1,324 mmt, then maize/corn at 721 mmt, then wheat at 627 mmt, and rice at 605 mmt.[13]

Cereal crops are amongst the most subsidized in the world. The European Union subsidizes agriculture to the tune of €48 billion per year and the United States $20 billion.[14] Coincidentally, the United States and European Union are the world's largest producers of grain.

By comparison, here are the numbers for the foods we recommend eating for your health, the foods humans have evolved to be able to consume naturally: All vegetables make up about 866 million metric tons a year, all fruits, 503 mmt; meat, 259 mmt; fish, 130 mmt; and eggs, 63 mmt. All of these combined still make up less than the total production of cereal crops alone.

Follow the money: governments and food manufacturers have invested in maximizing cereal production and exportation. If you currently believe that the grain recommendations on "healthy" eating charts promoted by the U.S. and U.K. governments have anything to do with your health, as opposed to, say, business reasons, then perhaps a rethink is in order.

If you are reading an original edition of our book years after its publication, it might be worth looking up current crop production figures. We imagine things will have only continued down this path.

Is There Anything Good about Cereal Grains?

So what is good about cereal grains? Well, they were a major factor of the agricultural revolution, which completely changed human society. Grains have enabled a massive explosion in population by supplying cheap, easily stored and transported energy. As we mentioned earlier, humans can survive on grains (for a time), although they are ultimately making us fat and unwell.

Grains freed us up from having to hunt and gather on a daily basis after their introduction to the human diet during the first agricultural revolution ten thousand years ago. This enabled human creativity to be focused on many divergent areas, which have ultimately led to the scientific, technological, and medical advancement of our species.

Perhaps now is the time where we can take stock and appreciate what grains have done for us, but also realize the damage they are currently doing to most of us. Initially, on an individual basis, we can make informed choices as to what we consume. It may be a case of going backward to go forward; our Paleolithic ancestors had it right in terms of nutrition for the health and well-being of the individual.

Over time, perhaps we can get society and governments to change their notions of nutrition and agricultural policy—we no longer need grain except for perhaps emergencies and in countries where there is a constant threat of famine. Of course, as a society, we would need to massively upregulate our production of livestock, fish, vegetables, fruits and so on. Is it worth it for our health and the sake of our children's health? We certainly think so.

The Story of a Modern Sweetener: High Fructose Corn Syrup

High fructose corn syrup was introduced into the food chain in the late 1970s and its use became widespread by the 1980s. Food manufacturers began using it because it is a cheaper sweetener, six times sweeter than sugar from sugar cane. Naturally occurring fructose is okay for us in very small quantities only in its natural form—notably whole fruit—and then that only accounts for around 5 percent to 10 percent of the weight of any fruit. High fructose corn syrup, however, is far from being natural.

Corn (maize) syrup in its initial state is pure glucose. To make high fructose corn syrup, manufacturers use enzymatic processing to convert the glucose into fructose. This fructose is then blended with regular corn syrup. The resulting product is a supersweet mix of both fructose and glucose.

High fructose corn syrup is then added to a vast array of processed foods; everything from soft drinks to cookies to ready meals. If you eat pre-prepared foods or drink soda, you are likely consuming a considerable amount of high fructose corn syrup every day.

A recent study, published in 2009, led by Kimber Stanhope of the Department of Nutrition, University of California, Davis, showed that human subjects put on a ten-week diet containing high amounts of fructose produced new fat cells around their heart, liver, and digestive organs. They also showed markers linked to diabetes and heart disease. This was over a short ten-week period; many people are consuming amounts of fructose similar to those used in this experiment every day of their lives.[15]

What was the reaction to this research from a spokesperson for the UK Food and Drink Federation? "It makes no sense to highlight one single ingredient as a cause of obesity."[16] If we were skeptics, we could say, of course it doesn't, if the companies you represent use that particular ingredient widely and indiscriminately.

What do the U.S. Food and Drug Administration have to say about high fructose corn syrup? Bear in mind that over 85 percent of the corn syrup produced in the United States is also of a genetically modified origin. Well, the FDA classifies high fructose corn syrup (HFCS) as generally recognized as safe (GRAS), not specifically recognized as safe though.

If 15 percent to 25 percent of our nutritional intake came from HFCS, as it does for many Americans, we'd like a bit more specificity about this matter. Especially about an ingredient that has only been in our food chain for the last thirty or so years (the fattest thirty years in the history of the human species).

The U.S. government subsidizes the production of domestic corn and places import tariffs on foreign sugar. Sucrose prices in America are amongst the (artificially) highest in the world. This, of course, makes HFCS the sweetener of choice for most U.S. food manufacturers and processors.

We tend to like buying the food we eat from local farmers whenever possible, preferably those who use more traditional farming methods. Can you imagine where the industrial production process for HFCS was developed?

It certainly wasn't your local farmer; it was, in fact, the Agency of Industrial Science and Technology Ministry of International Trade and Industry of Japan. As esteemed an establishment as it might be, the AISTMITIJ (for short) is not where we would choose to source 25 percent of our calorific intake from, whilst we still have a choice in the matter.

Studies have shown that increased consumption of fructose in particular and sugars in general is a causing factor of both obesity and insulin resistance.[17] Other research has found that soft drinks that contain HFCS can be up to ten times worse in terms of carbonyl compounds. These compounds are noted for causing diabetic complications like eye and nerve damage and foot ulcers.[18] Samples of HFCS have also been known to contain mercury.[19]

There have been a couple of studies which claim to show HFCS is no worse than table sugar. We need, however, to point out that the Corn Refiners Association, the American Beverage Institute, and Tate and Lyle (a large corn refiner) funded those studies.[20]

A key issue with HFCS is that it has led to a major increase in sugar consumption amongst the general population, by the back door, so to speak. It is hidden away in so many pre-packaged, manufactured foods and drinks that the majority of people are not aware that they are even consuming such a substance.

Although natural fructose is contained in small amounts in fruit, HFCS is not a natural product; it has to go through chemical synthesis to exist. HFCS is neither natural nor healthy. We would go so far as to say that HFCS has no place in the human diet whatsoever.

Bottom line: it is possible that regularly consuming foods and drinks containing HFCS will help you achieve tooth cavities, excess body fat, and potentially diabetes.

HFCS is a refined sugar, and we know that refined sugar is not healthy for us. HFCS is beyond refined; it is a chemically manufactured, cheap sugar substitute that serves the profiteers of the food industry and does nothing but potentially devalue our health as consumers.

Low-Calorie Artificial Sweeteners

It is common and understandable thinking to believe that by using low-calorie artificial sweeteners in place of sugars, we are doing a good thing for our weight loss goals.

This is the reason that many people looking to reduce their weight can be seen sipping on diet sodas or adding artificial sweeteners to their beverages, believing that because these sweeteners have zero or very low calorie counts, they will aid their fat loss progress.

There are a couple of issues with this. Firstly, many artificial sweeteners are unnatural chemical compounds that the human metabolism is not used to processing. Some of the artificial sweeteners on the market may even have long-term health ramifications.

Secondly, by continuing to consume sugar replacements, we are keeping our taste buds in training to desire unnaturally sweet foods. This ensures our addictive craving for refined carbohydrates and sugars remains, making long-term weight loss more challenging than it need be.

Artificial sweeteners may trick the mind and body into expecting and priming themselves to deal with high-calorie simple carbohydrates. In reality, they are getting the zero-calorie replacement, and this can actually stimulate our hunger for more food, as the body has not got what it was expecting.

A study published in *Behavioral Neuroscience*[21] found that rats who were given access to artificially sweetened liquid consumed a greater amount of calories from their regular food than rats that were just given sugared water.

A research project carried out at the University of Texas Health Science Center at San Antonio actually found that human subjects who drank diet soda were prone to gain more weight than those who drank regular soda.[22]

There are two main possible explanations for this, one being increased appetite stimulated by artificial sweeteners, the other being psychological. It is possible that people who drink diet sodas feel that they have been "good" by consuming a diet soda. They then go on to overeat other foods, believing that they have more leeway to do so because of their low-calorie soft drink consumption.

Some research has shown that artificial sweeteners trigger a similar increase in insulin levels as sugars. As we know, this increases appetite.[23]

For these reasons, we strongly advise avoiding all artificial sweeteners and products that contain them. If you are just beginning to follow our healthy diet and you are finding it a challenge to wait for your taste buds to adapt to your reduction in sugar intake, there are a couple of healthier options. We recommend the minimal use of a better natural sweetener, such as raw honey or real natural maple syrup. Do check the labels to ensure that no additional sugars have been added to your honey or maple syrup.

Over time, reduce the amount of honey or maple syrup you are using, ideally to a point where you don't use them at all, or only use them for occasional treats or special recipes, rather than allowing them to become a mainstay of your diet.

Modern and Future "Foods"

It is amazing, once you look past the tasty-looking photos on ready-meal packaging and processed foods, what ingredients you will actually find inside the box. One brand of shepherd's pie that we have looked at contains added maltodextrin, glucose syrup, lactose, *and* potato starch (maybe it was designed to be a shepherd's pie for those with an extremely sweet tooth!).

Interestingly, all four of those ingredients are carbohydrates or sugars, which food processors use as sweeteners, emulsifiers, and thickeners. Essentially, to disguise the fact that their food is not that tasty, they add forms of sugar to their products to sweeten and "improve" the taste. This tricks their customers' palates whilst letting them get away with selling what we consider to be very low-quality, low-cost ingredients (think maximum profit).

It seems that what we consume and what is being sold to us to consume within the mass market is becoming less and less like real food and more and more like an approximation of "food."

It is a good idea to keep in mind what the food manufacturers have in store for us in the future. It is highly likely that genetically modified foods will continue to be pushed on the consumer. In the United States, the Grocery Manufacturers of America already estimate that 75 percent of all processed foods contain a genetically modified ingredient.[24]

Our American and Canadian readers need to be aware that their countries do not require genetically modified foods or products containing genetically modified ingredients to be labeled as such. Slightly better news for our readers in the European Union and Australia is that GM foods do require labeling disclosing this information. Furthermore, in these countries, GM and non-GM foods must be kept separate throughout the entire production and processing chain.

Food manufacturers are also planning to bring "neutraceutical" products to a store near you. This is a "food" that works financially for the drugs and food industries, if not for the end consumer. A neutraceutical product is one where a highly processed food has synthetic vitamins and minerals added to it, so it can be sold under the guise of a "healthy" product. This already happens in the breakfast cereal market, where products are "fortified" with vitamins and minerals.

We'd like to point out that we think many of mankind's scientific developments have been wonderful in terms of labor saving and convenience—the car, the airplane, the computer, the Internet, to name but a few of the many that have benefited most of us.

However, when it comes to food, we believe Mother Nature truly knows best—if you go back to eating natural food which has been through either none or very minimal processing, you will be healthier.

Food manufacturers have tried to claim that the majority of additives they put into their products are preservatives. The reality is that about 90 percent of additives put into our food nowadays are "fake" or cosmetic; cheap, processed fats, refined starches, and refined sugars to boost the flavor and texture of poor quality starting ingredients.

The further we, as individuals, have become remote from the food production chain, the more ignorant we have become to what is happening to our food. Every now and again, a scare will occur and a consumer movement will raise awareness about a particular ingredient. The food industry may put their hands up and agree to ditch that particular ingredient, but there are hundreds more waiting in the wings that are equally distasteful and likely damaging to our long-term health. Keep your eyes and ears open, and ideally steer clear from all processed foods.

The Dangers of "Health" Foods

It is important to note that many products marketed as healthy products or sold in health food shops also contain poor quality ingredients. What often happens is a "health" product is sold on one or two of its ingredients that are assumed by the wider populace to be healthy—let's, for instance say, fruit and nuts.

We all tend to think that fruit and nuts are healthy, and the health food manufacturers rely on us being attracted to their product by the lead healthy ingredient. The vast majority of "healthy" fruit and nut bars, however, contain glucose syrup (or another sweetener) and vegetable oil.

In comparing a "healthy" fruit and nut bar and a well-known individual-sized chocolate bar, the so-called healthy bar had more total carbohydrates than the chocolate bar and roughly the same amount of sugar.

The issue we have with this is that someone who has decided to lose weight may swap her usual daily chocolate bar for one of these fruit and nut bars. She thinks that she is doing the right thing and that this "healthy" choice is going to help her lose weight.

However, in reality, she has swapped one bad food choice for another and is going to end up frustrated, thinking, "I've done everything right, I've got rid of the junk and started eating more healthily, and I still haven't lost weight."

Keep your eyes on the labels, even when you are buying foods that appear to contain some healthy ingredients. Many times, you will find that unhealthy ingredients or ingredients that are likely to ensure fat gain have been added and often even make up the majority of the so-called "healthy" product. When this is the case, steer clear; you are far better off consuming the natural foods nature provides, as outlined in *The ONE Diet.*

ଔ

In Conclusion:

- Stopping the consumption of refined carbohydrates helps to turn the body from fat-storage to fat-burning mode.

- To reduce body fat, most people need to consume fewer than 100 grams of carbohydrates a day, and the carbohydrates we do eat need to come from vegetables and fruit in our diet.

- Watch out for foods that are sold as "healthy" but actually contain grains and/or other unhealthy ingredients, and avoid artificial low-calorie sweeteners.

- Initially, when reducing carbohydrates, be prepared for short-term withdrawal symptoms. Break the sugar addiction and expect to lose around one to two pounds or 0.5 to one kilogram of body fat per week.

- Within a few weeks, your desire for sweet foods will naturally fade away.

- The original human diet as outlined in *The ONE Diet* is the antidote, a diet based on animal proteins and fats, vegetables and fruits.

Chapter 4.
The Power of Fats and Proteins

IN A NUTSHELL:

- Fats have been maligned by bad science, government agencies, the food industry, and the mass media. Saturated fats are in fact a great source of energy for our hearts and bodies. They are rich in energy and improve the functioning of the lungs, kidneys, our immune system, and cell membranes. Eating both fat and protein helps to decrease hunger and control appetite.

- Saturated fat is rich in important vitamins, notably A, D and K2, which aid the absorption of important minerals in our diet.

- We need a balance of omega-3 and omega-6 polyunsaturated fats. Most of us in the West get far too much omega-6, which is found in vegetable, grain and seed oils. Omega-6 has the effect of thickening the blood, whereas omega-3 thins the blood, reduces inflammation, and helps repair the body.

- Modern fats are not healthy for us; these include hydrogenated/partially hydrogenated fat, trans fats, interesterified fats (essentially a new type of trans fat), and fats/oils derived from vegetables, grains and seeds (the two exceptions to this rule are coconut oil and olive oil which are acceptable).

- Fat-free, low-fat, and reduced-fat processed foods and drinks are unnatural and are more likely to cause weight gain.

- Protein is vital for our health and weight loss goals. By far the best sources of protein are meat, game, eggs, fish and poultry.

- Legumes and pulses (mature beans and peas, including soybeans, lentils and peanuts) are poor sources of protein. They are usually best minimized in our diet.

ഗ

"The diet-heart hypothesis has been repeatedly shown to be wrong, and yet, for complicated reasons of pride, profit, and prejudice, the hypothesis continues to be exploited by scientists, fund-raising enterprises, food companies, and even governmental agencies. The public is being deceived by the greatest health scam of the century."

George Mann, ScD, MD,
Former Co-Director, The Framingham Study

Fats are the most maligned of the macronutrients, surrounded by misconception and unnecessary fears driven by government health departments, corporate profiteers, and often the mass media.

We could write a whole book on the damage done to the human diet and consequently our health by the misinformation surrounding fats. That has, however, already been done masterfully by Gary Taubes in *Good Calories, Bad Calories* (released in the United Kingdom as *The Diet Delusion*).

If you are interested in the full story behind the history of how fats came to be demonized and how far from the truth conventional thinking is (which is based on faulty science and an unproven hypothesis), we highly recommend reading *Good Calories, Bad Calories*.

Instead, in this book, we need to enable you to understand how many of the natural fats that have been demonized are actually some of the most health-giving foods you can eat and how crucial they are to your successful weight loss.

The first misconception we need to deal with is the most pervasive amongst the general public: the notion that the fat you eat directly becomes stored body fat.

If you consumed a diet of pure carbohydrate to excess, that carbohydrate can be stored as body fat; if you consumed a diet of pure protein to excess, that protein can be stored as body fat.

Whether it is protein, carbohydrate, or fat that you put into your system, what that energy starts out as does not dictate whether it gets stored as fat or not. Therefore, the fear that eating fat directly makes you store excess body fat is completely unfounded.

The needs and requirements of your body at any particular moment dictate what happens to any food type you eat. In a healthy individual, fat is being stored into cells and taken from cells to be used as energy all the time and at the same time. What is important to whether we get fatter or thinner is the net balance of this continually shifting equation.

When you eat dietary fat it may be used for your current energy needs, it may be used to make cell membranes or hormones, or it may be stored for later use. Similarly, protein or carbohydrates may be used as energy or converted to be stored as fat.

The fear that fat eaten can only make you fat is incorrect. The body has plenty of other uses for fat (and protein and carbohydrates) other than fat storage.

Here is the important take-home lesson: when you are eating healthily and have reduced or eliminated unhealthy refined carbohydrates, much of the energy in your diet will be derived from healthy fats.

Saturated fats are a good source of energy for your body to run on because they are rich in energy (9 calories per gram). When combined with an *appropriate* amount of protein and the right type of carbohydrates, you will not add excess body fat. Your current body fat will begin to drop as your body metabolizes its own fat stores for additional energy. In this environment (without excess refined carbohydrates stimulating hunger), it is actually quite difficult to consume too much fat.

For the vast majority of us, just by cutting out the unhealthy foods and eating the right foods as laid out clearly in *The ONE Diet*, we will lose our excess body fat. We will be able to do this without ever having to count calories or having to work out what percentage of our food is made up of fat, what percentage of protein, and what percentage of carbohydrates.

Saturated Fats

This brings us on to further major misconceptions about dietary fat, which are just as prevalent as the "eating fat makes you fat" fallacy. These misconceptions are that saturated fat and cholesterol are bad for your heart and your health. The vast majority of scientific research shows that saturated fat does not increase blood cholesterol and low-density lipoproteins, nor is it a cause of cardiovascular disease or a risk factor for heart disease.[1]

Saturated fats are actually critical to our health and well-being as they serve many important functions in our bodies. Saturated fats help the lungs and kidneys to function optimally; they reinforce our immune system, protect against diabetes, and aid our cell membrane receptors.

Our nervous system cannot function efficiently without saturated fats, and our most creative organ, the brain, is over 50 percent saturated fat. Saturated fat is also rich in crucial vitamins A, D, and K2. Overall, if any food type is deserving of the title "superfood," saturated fat certainly qualifies.

The work of Dr. Price and the Weston A. Price Foundation has shown that "in traditional diets, levels of these key nutrients (A, D, and K2) were about ten times higher than levels in diets based on the foods of modern commerce, containing sugar, white flour, and vegetable oil. Dr. Price referred to these vitamins as activators because they serve as the catalysts for mineral absorption. Without them, minerals cannot be used by the body, no matter how plentiful they may be in the diet."[2]

Natural saturated fats primarily found in animal products are a superb form of energy that our bodies have actually evolved to thrive on and are essential for both our long-term health and our immediate fat loss goals.

Healthy Sources of Saturated Fat

Butter

Ghee

Lard

Cheese

Eggs

Meat

Cream

Unrefined Virgin Coconut Oil

The reality is that fats are very healthy for you if you consume natural fats, the types of fat the human metabolism evolved to process naturally (full fat butter, full fat cream, animal fats, coconut oil, and so on) as opposed to modern, refined, and health-destroying fats (margarines; vegetable, grain and seed oils; and hydrogenated and artificial trans fats).

You will notice that coconut oil is the only non-animal source of saturated fat that we recommend here, as most plant oils consist primarily of polyunsaturated fats (which we will discuss later in this chapter). Coconut oil however contains over ninety percent saturated fats and therefore it is an excellent source of healthy saturated fats, along with the animal sources listed.

Nutrition Week reported in 1991 that regular consumers of margarine have twice the incidence of heart disease that butter eaters do.[3] A study published in the *Lancet*[4] shows that the fatty acids present in artery clogs are largely unsaturated (74 percent), of which 41 percent are polyunsaturated.

They found no link whatsoever between saturated fatty acids and aortic plaques. The very fat substitutes that the food manufacturers have marketed to us as healthy alternatives to natural fats are doing the real damage to our health.

Consider this: In "The Skinny on Fats,"[5] authors Enig and Fallon detail how between 1910 and 1970, consumption of animal fat decreased from 83 percent to 62 percent in the American diet. During the same timeframe, the amount of butter consumed dropped from eighteen pounds per person per year to just four pounds.

Yet levels of heart disease and obesity rose exponentially in the West during this same period. What has changed so dramatically about the modern Western diet during this period that can possibly account for this? Enig and Fallon point out consumption of refined vegetable oils and their derivatives have risen by a whopping 400 percent, and intake of sugar and processed foods in general has risen by 60 percent.

These are the very things that are alien to the human metabolism. There has been a massive decline in the use of traditional healthy saturated fats and a huge increase in food products that have no traditional, historic usage in human evolution and development.

We are then left with a general population struggling with their weight and health and fearful of the types of fat (natural saturated fats) that will actually improve their weight, health, and well-being.

Saturated fats are not bad for you; they are actually a form of energy on which the heart can thrive. They are so important to the heart that if we don't consume enough saturated fat in our diet, our bodies are stressed into making their own from carbohydrates and protein.

Cholesterol

Saturated fats' equally maligned partner, cholesterol, is chock-full of beneficial nutrients for human function. Cholesterol, a steroid metabolite, is an essential part of the structure of all of our cell membranes (this is true of every mammal, hence cholesterol's presence in animal products), and it is transported in our blood plasma.

Cholesterol has many important roles in the body, including ensuring appropriate membrane permeability, insulating neurons, aiding in the manufacture of steroid hormones, vitamin D, and bile acids, and metabolizing the fat-soluble vitamins.

Our livers can produce about 1,200 milligrams of cholesterol every day, auto-regulating, making more if our dietary intake of cholesterol is low and less if we intake a greater amount from our diet.

Cholesterol helps boost our immunity to infectious diseases, increases the strength of the intestinal wall, and, through its part in the manufacture of hormones, aids in the regulation of blood sugar and systemic inflammation. This type of inflammation is the primary factor in heart disease, and cholesterol actually helps to protect us from it. Interestingly, it is excess refined carbohydrates, excess vegetable, grain, and seed oils, and the artificial, man-made trans fats that are the main causes of this inflammation in the first place.

Dr. Kurt G Harris, MD,[6] points out that the best step we can take to avoid this inflammation and protect against atherosclerosis is to minimize the consumption of polyunsaturated fatty acids (found primarily in vegetable, grain, and seed oils), wheat, and excess sugars whilst at the same time consuming plenty of saturated fat.

Enter the Framingham Heart Study

Framingham is a town in Massachusetts, United States, with a population of around seventy thousand people. A unique medical/scientific study known as the Framingham Heart Study was initiated in Framingham in 1948 and is still ongoing today. Over fifteen thousand residents have taken part in the study so far, covering three generations of participants.

The purpose of the Framingham study is to "identify the common factors or characteristics that contribute to CVD (cardiovascular disease) by following its development over a long period of time in a large group of participants who had not yet developed overt symptoms of CVD or suffered a heart attack or stroke."[7]

The Framingham Heart Study has presented research on coronary heart disease, stating "total cholesterol was not associated with the risk of coronary heart disease."[8]

The overall findings at Framingham are perhaps best summed up by William Castelli, MD, a former director of the Framingham Heart Study:

"In Framingham, Massachusetts, the more saturated fat one ate, the more cholesterol one ate...the lower people's serum cholesterol.... We found that the people who ate the most cholesterol, ate the most saturated fat...weighed the least and were the most physically active." (1992)[9]

This is reinforced by renowned heart surgeon Michael DeBakey, MD, who states, "An analysis of cholesterol values...in 1,700 patients with atherosclerotic disease revealed no definite correlation between serum cholesterol levels and the nature and extent of atherosclerotic disease."[10]

Research published in the *Lancet* has shown that older people with high cholesterol outlive those with low cholesterol, primarily due to the benefit of cholesterol protecting against cancer and infections.[11]

Research carried out at the Yale University School of Medicine found that in subjects with low cholesterol readings, there were twice as many incidences of heart attack or death from a heart attack when compared to subjects with the highest cholesterol readings. They concluded that high cholesterol is simply *not* a risk factor for "all-cause mortality, coronary heart disease mortality, or hospitalization for myocardial infarction or unstable angina."[12]

Gary Taubes emphasizes the point in *Good Calories, Bad Calories* that nearly every scientific study that compares diet, cholesterol, and heart disease within a single population has failed to make any connection between eating saturated fats and cholesterol and heart disease.

You need not fear dietary cholesterol at all; in fact, the cholesterol in natural animal products such as meat, poultry, eggs, and cheese is both healthy and an important part of the human diet.

The dietary cholesterol to avoid is manufactured, powdered eggs, powdered milk, and any products that contain them. This is because the cholesterol in the majority of powdered eggs and milk has been oxidized in the manufacturing process, and oxidized fats are not good for our hearts. Stick with natural, health-giving sources of cholesterol.

The Polyunsaturated Fats: Omega-6 and Omega-3

The most common polyunsaturated fats in the human diet are omega-6 and omega-3. It is important that we have a balanced amount of omega-3 and omega-6 and not have a wide discrepancy between the two.

Typically, in Western, affluent countries, we consume far more omega-6 (largely from vegetable, grain, and seed oils) than omega-3 (found in foods like oily fish and meat from cattle raised on pasture).

Ideally, our consumption of omega-3 to omega-6 needs to be at a 1:1 ratio, but in westernized countries, this ratio can be out of whack by as much as 1:50! The problem with an imbalance favoring omega-6 is that it can thicken the blood and increase the risk of chronic diseases, including cardiovascular disease, and the potential risk for heart attack.

Omega-3, conversely, helps to thin the blood, reduce inflammation, and aids in the long-term repair of the body. The take-home lesson is simple: we need to reduce our consumption of omega-6-containing oils. This effectively means completely eliminating vegetable, grain, seed oils and products that contain them (with the exceptions of the previously mentioned unrefined virgin coconut oil which consists primarily of saturated fats and virgin or extra virgin olive oil, which is an acceptable oil rich in monounsaturated fat that we can use for dressing salads).

In other words we need to avoid oils such as sunflower, corn, soybean, safflower, canola, peanut, flaxseed, and products that contain them, which include most processed foods, mass-marketed mayonnaise, salad dressings, and fried foods (except those you fried in butter, ghee, or coconut oil).

Omega-3 oils, as mentioned, occur naturally in oily fish and meat.

With oily fish, there is a health concern due to the toxins they may contain because of the pollution levels in our oceans. The best types of fish with the typically lowest amount of toxins include salmon, tuna, anchovies, Atlantic herring, cod, Atlantic mackerel, sardines and trout.

With regards to cooking oily fish, it is necessary to cook slowly and gently, avoiding high heat; this will help preserve the healthy oils in the fish as much as possible.

Fact: Organic and pastured eggs also contain DHA (docosahexaenoic acid)/omega-3.

The benefits of a balanced intake of omega-3 and omega-6 fats include improved heart health, a healthy fatty acid balance within our cells, improved brain health and function, and improved protein synthesis after exercise. In addition to this, omega-3 has been shown to be beneficial in reducing prostate tumor growth and increasing survival rates. There are also links with reduced risk of breast cancer.

Simply by eliminating vegetable, grain, and seed oils from your current diet and consuming meat, pastured or organic eggs, and occasionally (once or twice a week) oily fish, too, your omega-3 to omega-6 ratio will be in a healthy balance.

The Bad News: Modern Fats

Artificial trans fats and hydrogenated fats are a completely modern phenomenon and only became a part of our diets from the 1900s onward, when companies began to use the hydrogenation technique to turn a liquid fat into a solid fat.

In hydrogenation, the original oil is heated to temperatures of up to 410 degrees Fahrenheit or 210 degrees Celsius in a high-pressure environment for as long as eight hours, whilst hydrogen gas is injected. During this process, tiny particles of copper or nickel are added which destroy the good essential fatty acids, replacing them with trans-fatty acids.

These companies found they could turn cheap vegetable oils into hydrogenated and partially hydrogenated solid fats, at a profit. The apparent consumer "benefits" were margarines that, unlike natural butter, would spread straight from the fridge and have a longer shelf life, prolonging the period before rancidity would set in compared with natural butter.

Hydrogenated oils for frying also have a longer fry life, and hydrogenated fats give food a particular texture that is considered advantageous by fast food companies. Food manufacturers use hydrogenated/partially hydrogenated oils in their recipes due to their low cost, their convenience, and the fact that they increase the shelf life of their products.

The amount of trans fats in hydrogenated fat varies from 1 percent in fully hydrogenated vegetable oil to as great as 60 percent in partially hydrogenated oils. The amount of trans fats present is dependent on the degree to which the oil has been hydrogenated.

Look out for these fats on food labels and avoid:

Hydrogenated fat

Partially hydrogenated fat

Vegetable fat

Vegetable oil

Vegetable margarine

Vegetable shortening

All oils made from vegetables, grains, or seeds (with the exceptions of unrefined virgin coconut oil and olive oil).

Artificial, man-made trans fats are the worst type of fats for us and have no place in the human diet. It is artificial trans fats that can increase people's risk of coronary heart disease by increasing levels of low-density lipoprotein cholesterol and reducing levels of high-density lipoprotein cholesterol in our bodies, putting our cholesterol levels out of balance.

Recent studies have shown that artificial trans fats increase the risk of coronary heart disease more than any other food type and are estimated to be responsible for up to one hundred thousand deaths per year in the United States alone.[13] Let's make this clear: artificial trans fats are to be avoided if we care about our health.

The Case Against Artificial Trans Fats Expanded

Research studies have been coming in over the last few years confirming just how bad artificial trans fats are for us. They have been connected to prostate cancer and greater risk of breast cancer. French research has suggested the risk of breast cancer may be increased by 75 percent by an increased intake of trans fats.[14]

In terms of obesity, there appears to be a link between trans fats and increased weight, specifically abdominal fat. This has been demonstrated in a six-year experiment on monkeys. One group was fed natural monounsaturated fat and the other group trans fat; both diets contained a similar number of calories. Over the six-year period, the trans-fat-fed monkeys gained 7.2 percent of their body weight whilst their monounsaturated counterparts only gained 1.8 percent.[15]

Artificial trans fats are now being implicated as a likely cause of liver dysfunction, as they are metabolized differently in the liver than natural fats and interfere with a vital enzyme, delta 6 desaturase. Artificial trans fats have also been found to cause inflammation, atherosclerosis, diabetes, obesity, and general immune system dysfunction.[16]

The problem is our bodies cannot recognize the artificial trans fats and don't know how to process them, so they get absorbed through our cell membranes and wreak havoc with the metabolism of the cells. This may be caused in part by the fact that the hydrogenation process actually changes the placing of hydrogen atoms in the fatty acid chain.

So why are trans fats put in processed foods in the first place? That question is simple to answer: the trans fats are cheaper and have a longer shelf life, which suits the food manufacturers and retailers even if it doesn't suit your body and health.

Incidentally there are naturally occurring trans fats in some animal products, these are only present in trace amounts and are perfectly healthy for us to consume. It is artificial trans fats that we need to avoid.

Interesterified Fats

We need to break it to you: things are getting somewhat worse in the mass-market food industry rather than better. As more and more consumers are cottoning on to the fact that artificial trans fats are to be avoided at all costs, the food manufacturers are not sitting on their laurels and just accepting defeat, they've got new plans for our food supply.

Introducing…interesterified fats. Sound interesting? The all-new, "improved," chemically modified, interesterified fats are here. Yes, they still have the long shelf life; yes, they are still hydrogenated; and yes, the fat molecules are still unnaturally rearranged.

It's an old "enemy" returned with a makeover and an as-yet-untarnished or at least unrecognized name that may slip past those scanning the nutritional information on food packaging.

Our advice remains the same as for artificial trans fats: avoid at all costs. Especially as research on these new fats suggests they may be even worse for us than trans fats, having the ability to alter human metabolism and raise blood sugar levels to an even greater degree.[17]

We were unable to find any long-term studies carried out on the health of human subjects placed on a diet containing interesterified fats. It would be most wise to ensure that your food does not contain this artificially manufactured fat.

They Tried to Make Us Eat Low Fat and Fat Free

By now you will know that it is grains, refined carbohydrates, and sugars, and the food products that contain them, that drive weight gain. You will also have grasped that the traditional natural fats are what our bodies have evolved to thrive on. You will have understood that eating fat does not cause fat storage. In fact, calories we eat from fat or any other macronutrient can usually only be converted into body fat if we consume too much grain and and added sugars.

This brings us to fat-free and low-fat products, which are heavily promoted by the food manufacturers and retailers. These products are a con. The food industry realized a long time ago that that people are irrationally scared of the word "fat". This irrational fear is an easy mistake to make *if* a person does not know the science behind the foods we eat. To the layperson, the thinking goes, "When I eat fat, that fat must end up becoming a part of the fat on my body."

The food industry knowingly exploits this error in the common perception of nutritional fat. Therefore, they bring to the market a "new" breed of food, untested for the long-term effects on us, with the very ironic labels "fat free" and "low fat."

Ironic, because to make up for removing the natural fats from these products, the fat content has been sacrificed for a greater percentage of carbohydrate content in the overall macronutrient breakdown of the product.

It is refined carbohydrates and sugar that drive unhealthy weight gain. By removing the natural fat and thereby replacing it with carbohydrate, you end up with a product that is far more likely to make a person fat and stimulate increased hunger. Of course, stimulating increased hunger may well benefit food manufacturers and retailers, if not your waistline and wallet.

Bottom line: steer well clear of processed foods that claim to be fat free and low fat—they have been doctored away from being natural and contain a greater percentage of ingredients that are likely to cause weight gain.

Protein

Protein is a very important component of our overall nutrition and is not surrounded by as much misinformation as the other macronutrients, fats and carbohydrates.

There are about twenty amino acids in protein, at least eight of which are considered essential amino acids and must come from our diet. The eight essential amino acids are isoleucine, leucine, lysine, threonine, tryptophan, methionine, histidine, and valine.

Our protein requirements are best met by consuming sources of protein such as meat, poultry, eggs, and fish. Meat contains all the essential amino acids.

When purchasing meat, look at the packaging to see what the animals have been fed. Grass-fed animals will provide a somewhat healthier meat than those that have been fed a diet of grain. Meat from grain-fed animals will have a higher ratio of omega-6 fat, whereas those fed grass will have a higher amount of omega-3 fats.

Protein Requirements

The vast majority of people will adequately meet their protein needs by eating between 8–16 ounces (250–500 grams) of animal foods (meat, poultry or fish) per day.

By following The ONE Diet, your protein intake will be very close to optimal without ever having to count grams of protein or meat. We suggest it is psychologically healthier to avoid obsessing about gram counts or calorie counts and besides for the vast majority of us, it is unnecessary anyway.

The Value of Red Meat

Red meat is beneficial for both the heart and the nervous system and contains valuable coenzyme-Q10, vitamins B12 and B6, carnitine and zinc. Additionally, the saturated fat and cholesterol in red meat is an excellent and health-promoting source of energy.

A further plus point to protein consumption in general is that when metabolized, protein releases glucagon, which is known to decrease hunger and helps to control appetite.

New Research Shows How Long Humans Have Been Eating Meat

A very recent archaeological find has shown that our ancestors were eating meat almost a million years earlier than previously had been thought. The study led by Zeresenay Alemseged of the California Academy of Sciences and published in the journal *Nature* in 2010 details that animal bones discovered in Ethiopia show cut marks from stone tools used to scrape off meat and the bones themselves broken open to extract the marrow (a fantastic source of fat). These bones have been dated to 3.4 million years ago.

This helps to remind us that meat and animal fat are foundational to our natural ancestral human diet.

What about Legumes and Pulses?

Legumes and pulses include soybeans, mature beans and peas (including dried beans and peas), alfalfa, lentils, and peanuts.

When aiming to reduce body fat, we recommend avoiding consuming legumes for several reasons. As many vegetarians know, legumes contain some protein (the amount and quality of the protein is variable depending on the type of legume). However, they typically have quite a high carbohydrate content that may slow or even halt weight loss if consumed regularly.

Now while this carbohydrate content won't cause the same problems as some other sources of carbohydrates (cereal grains, for example). They still contain a relatively high proportion of carbohydrate, which may add considerably to your daily carbohydrate intake.

The major point is that there are healthier and more digestible sources of the nutrients found in legumes, in other foods that we recommend. It makes little sense to add legumes to your diet, especially whilst you are focusing on losing weight.

Additionally, the bioavailability of minerals in legumes may be relatively low—in effect, the body has somewhat of a hard time digesting legumes. This is the reason many legumes must be soaked in water and drained before being cooked.[18]

This of course doesn't completely preclude them from making an occasional appearance in your eating habits, especially once you have obtained your goal weight and particularly if you really enjoy them. Just know there are far healthier choices for all the nutrients found in legumes in meat, fish, eggs, and vegetables.

It is worth mentioning that edible immature beans and peas, many of which can be eaten in their pods, are however healthy and perfectly acceptable on The ONE Diet, including: green beans, french beans, runner beans, string beans, green peas, snap peas, sugarsnap peas, mangetout and snow peas. Use these peas and beans as you would vegetables.

Avoid Modern Soy Products

The traditional soy products consumed by Asians, like miso, tempeh, and tamari, for example, are fermented, and this natural process makes the soy safe to consume. Modern, westernized soy products, protein, and meat substitutes, however, are far from being a healthy food source, and have been implicated in depressing thyroid function and blocking mineral and protein absorption.[19]

Furthermore, soy protein cannot be considered a complete protein, as it is deficient in both methionine and cystine. Modern processing of Western soy products also often denatures the amino acid lysine, which means that even if you put the negative health consequences of consuming soy to one side it is still far from being an ideal or complete source of protein.

So if you are going to occasionally eat soy, ensure it is one of the traditional Asian fermented varieties and not a meat substitute, a protein powder, or any other unusual modern concoction.

ㆍ

IN CONCLUSION:

- By consuming natural fats like full fat butter, ghee, lard, full fat cream, cheese, eggs, animal fats, and coconut oil, and *avoiding* vegetable, grain, and seed oils, margarines, hydrogenated/partially hydrogenated fats, and trans fats, we revert to eating as nature intended.

- For optimal health, we need to consume both saturated fats and unsaturated fats as provided by The ONE Diet.

- Avoid all processed foods that are marketed as fat free, low fat, or reduced fat.

- Whenever you can, purchase meat and eggs from animals that have been raised on pasture rather than grain.

- Avoid modern/Western soy products like fake "meat" and soy protein powders.

Chapter 5.
Our Minds May Make Us Fat

IN A NUTSHELL:

- The mindset, perspective, and attitude we adopt affect our experience and our reactions. The way we communicate with others and, more importantly, with ourselves can have a massive impact on our life experience.

- Our psychology requires close examination if we are to avoid being trapped by historical continuity. The tendency is to continue doing what we have always done, what's known, and what we have become accustomed to.

- Many are trapped by past traumas and events, such as childhood bullying, which result in weight gain. Boredom and loneliness can also result in some of us eating excessively just to fill time and distract us from pain.

- Some of us may have developed "Why should I do what they tell me" or "I don't care" attitudes, even if they are not in our best interest. This type of self-destructive behavior and self-sabotage can lead to serious long-term damage.

- The internal dialogue (how and what we say to ourselves) and our spoken words impact on our actions—be aware of what you are saying to yourself and others.

- Seeking to fit in and be part of a group often results in adopting attitudes and habits that are contrary to our best interest. The cost of "fitting in" can have a very high price tag. Additionally, it can also elevate our stress levels and, consequently, negatively impact our lives.

- In essence, though, it is our beliefs that determine what we experience in our lives. Our beliefs (programming) about our self-image perpetuate our shape and size. These programs have been instilled by others and adopted by us as if they are true. Few challenge the origins of beliefs born in our childhood.

- We are driven by our emotions. These tend to be the pursuit of pleasure or the avoidance of pain. Pain is mostly evidenced as fear, whereas pleasure is evidenced as joy. By becoming aware of our current habits surrounding food, nutrition, and eating, we can ensure we are serving our goal; otherwise, they will need to be constructively changed.

- The tendency is to experience emotions before our mind has had a chance to think through a situation. Once an emotion has been felt, we are blinded to other possibilities. This results in our forgoing the need to think something through and explore other perspectives.

- Some of us may have developed obsessive behaviors, addictions, and compulsions around food. These will need to be addressed. In some cases, seeking professional help may be beneficial.

ᴄ꙰

Let's start with the most subtle psychological trap. Some people will find it easy to fall into a psychological cause that would allow them to continue the use of fattening foods. If, as you read through the possible psychological reasons for having excess fat, you find something that resonates strongly with you, then we would suggest you seek out a professional who can help you move on.

We need to understand that the additional weight we may be carrying could be as a result of some underlying cause. It could be as simple as a lack of understanding of nutrition, a sort of comfortable naivety that ensures we get plenty of oral gratification. It could be that we are insecure and need to be seen as big; it could be that it is the only way we have found of getting attention.

It may also be that the weight on, weight off pattern is what we have become accustomed to spending most of our time dealing with. That it is, in effect a big element of our daily lives, we are consumed with food and everything related to food.

CHILDHOOD ISSUES CAN DRIVE OUR ADULT BEHAVIOR

Case Study

How Weight Gain Can Be Psychologically Driven

The mind, in its need for self-preservation, will do just about anything to survive. Some years back a client came for assistance to help her lose fat weight. She was in her thirties and just could not get the fat off her body.

This affected not only her body weight, her posture, and her general energy levels; it also affected the relationships that she sought. We say "sought" because it was rare for her to be in a relationship and, more often than not, it would be with someone who was otherwise committed, a married man or the like.

It is not easy finding someone when your size erodes your confidence and, what's worse, intimidates the other person. The tendency is to wait and hope that someone has had a few drinks too many and is left over at the bar. A way is found to justify the sleepover, and in the morning it is awkward, so they carry on as if nothing happened. You get the picture.

The question that needed answering was simple. What purpose is the excess fat serving for this woman? What was it that prevented her from getting to her comfortable weight? We used a process called Gold Psychotherapeutic

Counseling to help open up her mind to the cause of her excess.

The process revealed that it was unsafe to be of normal size. This would attract unwanted attention. Her belief was that the fat that she was carrying was her protection. It kept her safe from being hurt and humiliated. The very thing she feared was the very thing that was happening to her.

To get to the cause was vital, as only it can set the mind free from its misconceptions. Once understood and worked through, a moment of liberating enlightenment occurred. Suddenly it all made perfect sense. Historic continuity stopped and a new dawning occurred.

The situation for this young woman was quite upsetting. As a child aged around six, she was encouraged to sit on the lap of an old man, who then inappropriately touched her. She did her best to avoid the situation by sticking her belly out as far she could to make it difficult for him. Nonetheless, she found herself trapped by him.

The more she stuck her belly out, the harder it was for the man to reach her private parts. As time progressed, she found herself developing a stomach that was so wide that no person could physically put his or her hands around her.

For almost three decades, her mind kept her safe from anyone getting close to her. When we considered the side effects of such an event, it was a catalogue of self-destructive acts for the benefit of self-preservation.

Many beliefs developed that debilitated her weight loss from happening. In order to be safe, she needed to make herself big. That was the priority: just get big, because if she was big, then she was safe.

The event also left her feeling ashamed of what had happened. In adulthood, it manifested as feelings of guilt. So she understood why, when she sneaked that extra burger and never told anyone, she perpetuated her feelings of guilt. It was, after all, her "guilty secret."

For this woman, the realization, shocking as it was, was enough for her to work out that the incident was more than just about food. It affected her opinion of men generally in the sense that she had given birth to the idea that men were strong and dirty and only wanted one thing.

Once the debriefing and reframing was completed, she was able to get on with life. As a point of interest, although her body weight and size altered to some degree, she was still on the larger side of average. This, though, no longer caused her to be distressed. Food was no longer used to numb her fear, and she has been able to find a partner who wants to spend time with her.

Bullying

Where bullying has been a problem in childhood, it can manifest in adulthood as an eating disorder. If we are in an environment where we feel threatened or suffer physical or emotional abuse, it is possible to develop a belief that our size will protect us. This is especially so where the abuser was also perceived as big. A thought may develop that suggests that if we too are big, then we are safe, or that if we are big, then we may not be a target for bullies.

The fear of attack is ever present in the mind of a victim. There are many ways to react to this type of situation. For example, we might develop sufficient wealth to have a wall of money around us; we might acquire a physique that makes us powerful; we may even attach ourselves to someone or a group that we perceive as being protective of us. We may even develop a following to keep us safe. The development of strategies to cope is necessary for our survival.

Being constantly put upon during school by boys that sought to be seen as tough, or having the pretty girls make us feel ugly, can result in some terrible if not tragic outcomes. Things that were said or not said can scar our mind in ways that are almost unbelievable.

There are many such examples, and it would take another book to deal with this subject fully. Suffice it to say that bullying has consequences later in life. The effect of bullying is serious and needs to be dealt with by a professional.

Principally this book is for those who have simply become fat through eating the wrong foods and feel uncomfortably large. The key word in this is "uncomfortable." Take time to ponder on the subject of your emotions. What happens when you simply do not pay attention to your diet and nutrition? Take time to ponder this question if you want to be free of the excess weight that you carry.

Comfort Eating

Food is used by the body to nourish and energize our system, enabling us to function and survive. It has a very close association with another ingredient in our formative years between birth and age two, that being nurture. We are mostly fed in the warm comfort of a mother's arms. Safe, secure, orally gratified with warm nourishment and a feeling of being loved and cared for.

For some people, it's a place our mind remembers well— not necessarily conscious memories, rather a recognizable feeling. It is a psychological place we may want to go to when things are not going well for us. Our mind can transport us there in an instant. All we need do is immerse ourselves in flavors, textures, and smells that fulfill our needs for comfort.

The phrase "comfort eating" has been around for many years, to the point where it has lost its significance. Perhaps it can be better understood if we give a better explanation as to the mechanism that kicks in when we are stressed, under duress, or, worse still, distressed.

When things are not going as well as we would like them, we might just shrug off the situation and get on with our day. When, though, we are under duress or feeling distressed, we are likely to seek gratification, and the fastest way to accomplish this is to feed our pain with pleasure.

Case Study

A concerned mother sought assistance for her daughter, who was sixteen at the time and who was having some difficulties. It appears that she was consuming large quantities of up to forty-eight cans of cola per week. If she did not get her drink, she would become angry, then withdraw from her parents and lock herself in her room. This young woman was distraught and confused as to why her mother brought her for help, as she felt there was no problem.

After an initial assessment, it seems that she was preparing for her exams and was under a great deal of pressure to pass. She was encouraged to talk through the feelings that preceded her need to indulge and revealed that she believed the cola eased her anxiety.

Once she had expressed her emotions fully, she was encouraged to reflect on where her memories took her when she had her first experience of cola. This simply required a quiet, still mind and time to allow the mind to reflect.

She then recalled a time when her parents had bought her a kitten. She was about four years old and loved the new addition to the family. Her recollection took her to a time when, while playing with the kitten, she received a swipe from the cat's claws that was very painful.

She was scratched on her arm and screamed out loud in pain. Her mother came in, lifted her up, and attempted to comfort her. She took her into the kitchen and said, "Have some cola and it will all be better."

It sounds ludicrous to imagine that the mind would continue to use this as a future fix to painful experiences. The sugar content would have certainly caused a distraction. What her mind did was to use that experience for future fixes. Comfort is sought whenever we feel distressed.

Childhood Programming

It is not unusual to hear parents say, "If you are a good girl, we can go for a burger and fries and you can choose your own milk shake." How's that for programming? We never stood a chance. Now we associate being good with eating this type of burger, fries, and milk shake.

This child is being programmed to eat more than she needs to. That child one day becomes an adult and continues to overorder. Often we find that we continue a pattern of overindulgence.

The guilt factor is a big one when it comes to overeating. How some parents use guilt defies logic in such a way that it can leave us speechless. Imagine how our mind is manipulated when we are told that we should think ourselves lucky that there is food on our plate whilst there are so many poor people around the world starving. So we are now not feeling good at the thought of leaving food and uncomfortable when we have overfilled our belly.

In some instances, we are told that if we do not behave ourselves, we will go without food. A punishment is then associated with the denial of food. Is it any wonder that we so easily learn that ultimately the only thing that we can control is what we eat? That it is used as a reward and as a punishment? There are implications of this to anyone who has been hurt in childhood and has learned that he can control his, and occasionally others', degree of pleasure or pain.

Some people even develop disorders such as bulimia and anorexia when they reach an emotional impasse and perceive themselves unable to control the outcome of some event. That they need to take control of something is obvious through their actions. It is perhaps the only emotional vent available to them which provides both pain and pleasure.

Under certain circumstances, it is possible to find ourselves driven to self-destruction by a situation that we have little or no control over. For instance, we might discover that the only times we get any attention from our parents or carers is when we are doing something inappropriate.

If we begin to realize that all eyes are upon us when we have put too much food in our mouth, we might notice that suddenly we are told not to do that, and then observed to see if we are still doing it. We might notice that the attention stops when we have conformed to the request to stop stuffing our mouth.

It may be that in that moment, we do it again—we stuff our mouth and suddenly the attention is back on us, and probably with more intensity. Quickly, we have learned to get attention by pigging out. "If you eat like that you will get fat" just adds to the attention and points us in the direction that we are going.

If we sense that we are a source of shame to our family and we stick out and get noticed while our parents are reeling in embarrassment, this may add to our satisfaction. We have found a way to get attention and cause discomfort, at least, or pain, at best, to those who are not appreciating us. This may also add to our own lack of self-appreciation.

It may be that we feel bad about ourselves and lacking in self-worth, we decide to punish ourselves by overindulging and perpetuating our distorted appearance year in, year out. It appears that when we get the bit between our teeth and decide to prove to everyone that we are going to do what we are going to do, things can go horribly wrong. We self-destruct by abusing our body's ability to regulate digestion and swell to evidence our success.

Once we are carrying too much weight, we are caught in a trap of our own making. We have adopted new habits and behaviors that are going to be challenging to alter.

Being witness to children who have been scolded for not eating what is put on their plate is unpleasant. Common sense seems to be in short supply for some. Not all children are destined to be mammoth eaters. In most cases, if we just follow a tasteful and naturally benefiting nutritional diet, we are doing what is best for our children and their long-term survival.

What Does Our Size Achieve for Us?

On the subject of attention, it would be prudent to ponder on how much attention we are getting being the size we are. Does it fit in with an image we have grown up with? There are those who have grown up being known and referred to as "big guy." It could be that a name or attitude has been used to label a person and his or her size has been implied in that label.

We need to be conscious of all the details that refer to our size. Everything from "Mary sits in the big chair" to "Give the big portion to Jackie." From clothes that people might buy for us to the chocolate box for a treat, all these actions go towards our developing an attitude about our body and how we believe we are perceived.

Attention is as necessary as food for the vast majority of people.

Case Study

A client who came to lose weight because she could not receive in vitro fertilization (IVF) treatment until she reached an acceptable weight discovered that her mind was keeping weight on for her protection. At the age of eleven, she had an elder sister who was pregnant and just disappeared one day, never to be seen again.

Through dealing with her core beliefs, she had discovered that she had developed a belief that if you are with child, you disappear. It appears that in that South American country at the time, thousands of people were disappearing. Her sister was one of those people. The client was the last family member to see her alive.

A belief developed that if you are pregnant, you disappear. Her body adapted sufficiently so as to make pregnancy very difficult. The underlying cause of her weight gain was a protection for her. Once the debriefing occurred and treatment was completed, she went on to have two children.

Modeling

Much learning occurs through a process called modeling. Modeling is similar to copying or mimicking another person's behavior, characteristics, or mannerisms. This is often obvious when we watch children emulate their parents' behavior toward their younger sibling. A child that has a finger wagged in his or her face is then likely to do the same to a younger sibling.

The way we survive is dependent on watching what our elders (people that we perceive as being better than we are) do, and do not do, and incorporating this into our repertoire. A child is developing programs through being instructed and by modeling others. Watching Dad receive the largest portion is likely to instill the belief (pattern) that the male eats more that the others.

Being told that we are this or that is another way of programming our young minds. "You are so greedy" is highly likely to result in us fulfilling that belief once the idea is accepted. Why would it not be accepted if the person that has brought us onto the planet tells us so? He or she would not lie to us.

What is key to remember is that once we have learned something, it is not so easy to unlearn it. It appears that once a pattern of behavior has been established and therefore taken root in our psyche, it becomes absorbed into our operating system and becomes part of who we know to be us.

Modeling does not just stop at behaviors; it goes on to affect other attributes, such as body size and appearance. In many ways, we become what we focus on. Our most dominant thoughts guide our perception and, consequently, our behavior.

THE MIND AND PATTERNS OF BEHAVIOR THAT MAY BE KEEPING YOU OVERWEIGHT

Boredom

Boredom is a covert and extremely dangerous condition to be suffering from. Boredom can result in all manner of symptoms which more often than not result in overeating. The symptoms of boredom are many and varied; some people can take up sports, which bring them close to death in order to feel alive, whilst others are able to maintain an illicit relationship for years, to add to their uneventful life.

If we do not do something to ensure that our life has some meaning, then it is likely to result in feelings of discomfort at one end of the scale and outright rage at the other, need to do something to be free of this feeling, which, if unchecked, can become a dangerous and unpredictable threat to our being.

Mostly people get around it by developing hobbies that may not mean much to most of us but that satisfy a great need to the hobbyist. Collecting train numbers might be a great pastime for one person; another may fill his or her life with magazines that talk about other people's accomplishments. Mostly the television has many people mesmerized sufficiently to entertain their needs whilst selling them what to buy next.

For some, none of these things will fulfill that hollow feeling inside. They need some oral gratification when faced with nothing to do. So, into the freezer and in front of the TV to start eating a quart of ice cream or something similar to pass away the time and get engrossed in the seductive flavors and a fantasy reality.

Perhaps boredom is one of the most unrecognized sources of disease to humanity. We are, to a lesser or greater degree, capable, at the flick of a switch, of doing something crazy and then later regretting having done it. The issue of boredom needs to be addressed as a matter of priority in our endeavors to reduce fat.

Ensuring that we are fully and meaningfully occupied is critical to our survival. This goes far beyond weight loss; it includes all areas of our life. It is prudent to ponder on the activities that bring about fulfilling experiences. Do not underestimate the importance of this. Just think: in the past, what has happened to you at times of great boredom?

Do you find yourself behaving erratically or spontaneously at times and regretful of your actions? Be aware of this and design a way forward for your weight control that includes a meaningful activity. If it happens to include some physical activity and movement, all the better.

Loneliness

Loneliness is equally painful for many and does have some similarities with boredom in the sense that comfort eating is almost the norm. The problem with loneliness is that the sufferer tends to suffer in silence or, conversely, behaves desperately in an attempt to seek attention.

There are a number of reasons for this, most of which arise from childhood. If we were denied affection in our childhood, then we are likely to crave it in our adulthood. If we are unable to interact with others appropriately, then we are left with a craving and an abundance of food to choose from and feed on to compensate.

Our Minds Hear Everything We Say: What We Tell Others We Also Tell Ourselves

Our mind does not easily differentiate between saying something and believing that it is not meant, and saying something and meaning it. Someone eating an ice cream or a supersized double burger and saying with a flippant attitude to his friend, "I don't care, I just want it," is putting himself at risk and could seriously jeopardize his progress.

Our mind, as explained in other sections of this book, is easily duped. It hears anything and everything that we say and looks to implement our suggestion. Just think that when we talk of another, we are talking to ourselves at the same time.

You could almost hear the response if the mind was to be engaged in dialogue. "I don't care, I just want it" may have the response of "OK, this is what we do now." In little or no time, we look to get into our clothes and realize that we have overindulged and start getting frantic about getting the fat off.

Our mind is focused on what we say and where our attention is placed. It does not reason without your consent and engagement. It does not challenge unless you instigate a challenge. Our beautiful mind simply says "yes" to everything we say.

Self-suggestions, such as "this is going to be hard," result in our mind agreeing and perceiving that it will be hard and then experiencing it as hard.

If the next sentence we might think is "it's going to be easy," our mind simply agrees with everything we say. It is a "yes" mechanism.

Defiance

The defiant eater is one who knows that what she is doing is not good for her yet continues to overindulge simply on the basis of "Why shouldn't I." The "I don't care" attitude that defiant eaters perpetuate in company may not be quite the same when they are in the privacy of their own space. If you are struggling with your weight and believe that this could be you, then caution. Weeks of perseverance can be undone in minutes if we are not vigilant and thoughtful of our greater good.

Self-destruction is a serious issue when considering weight loss. Could it be that we are so angry that we have a "Frack it!" attitude on one hand and an "Enough already!" on the other? Could it be that something in our past still controls us to some degree? A poisonous attitude could be undoing our progress.

Peer Pressure

What's popular isn't always what right and what's right isn't always what's popular. Just because the masses are into a particular drink—you know, a superskinny, half-fat, supersoft, extra mocha, double bubble, vanilla-laced special—does not mean that it's necessarily going to be good for you. What it might mean is that you fit in with the crowd, you are normal in your social circle. You are accepted as hip and trendy, and you are likely to love it. But then you would; it's addictive in two respects, the need to fit in and the sugar rush.

In this day and age, with chemists able to refine scents and create aromas and flavorings capable of tricking our minds and convincing us that something smells great and tastes good, it is not easy to trust just the nose as we may have done in the past. We need facts that stand up to scrutiny and are in keeping with nature's laws.

It is easy to comply and to fit in; after all, the opportunities are abundant and the service is impeccable. We walk into the sandwich bar and find it difficult to resist someone saying to us, "The usual?" We enjoy the recognition, the feeling that we are someone special.

Perception and Pressure

Perception is a kind of translation mechanism. What the mind does with what it sees is perception.

It is a natural and normal thing for the mind to protect itself as best it can whenever and wherever it perceives itself under threat. The mind protects itself by ensuring that at times of threat; it increases its resources to the maximum that it is capable.

There is historic evidence that wherever a war occurs, the procreation levels increase phenomenally once the war is over. It is human nature to fight extinction. We are programmed to keep hold of life for as long as we can, and when threats occur, we need to build reserves.

We expect some to say, "But wait, I am not at war, and therefore I do not need to increase resources." Well, to some degree, you are right; you are not necessarily at war, but you may experience the same emotional states that a person at war may experience. By this, we mean that although you are not fighting a battle, you are fighting to be safe.

The possibility of losing your job or being left alone, of having no money or friends, of not belonging, causes stress and anxiety not dissimilar to that felt in battle. Different place, same symptoms.

As we grow into adulthood, we develop attitudes known as "absurd magical beliefs" (AMB). These allow us to cope with fears and anxieties that occasionally occur. In some instances and where the level of fear is extended, these can manifest in our adult life as obsessive or compulsive traits.

What can happen when we, as children, are going through a tough time is that we find a way of temporarily allaying our fears. This is accomplished by allowing our imagination to focus on something different, something away from where we are.

As children, we might on the way home from school tap every third post in the railings, or look to walk on a section of wall, or even avoid walking on the cracks on the pavement. Should we fail by slipping off the wall or stepping on a crack, we might start again from the beginning where time permits.

This is the mind's way of distracting our attention away from something painful toward something else. So long as we are consumed by that something else, it works.

Most people seek to avoid pain where possible. When we speak of pain, we are talking about emotional pain that often is not evidenced by others. Emotional hurt can take many forms and be caused by a multitude of reasons.

The shattering of a relationship, the loss of a loved one, losing a job, and similar situations can cause us to feel helpless or see the situation as hopeless. Where we are not able to find a solution, we are likely to utilize an emotional stabilizer to ease the pain.

We might rally support from family and friends, or we might behave dramatically to be heard and noticed to have some attention given to us. Often we simply head for the fridge.

Fear, Greed, and Gluttony

We as human beings have, to a lesser or greater degree, addictive personalities. Once we have something we like, we want it again, we want it more, and we develop an ever-increasing appetite for it. We want to own it. We are attracted to all things we enjoy and yet fear loss. We fear losing our youth, our partner, our friends, our lovers, our money, our power, etc.

It is important to explore an area critical to taking back control of how and what we experience in our lives. We are all driven by a combination of fear and greed. It is important at this stage to define and differentiate between greed and gluttony.

Greed simply means more. "I want more time to swim; it is something I enjoy and want more of." When we enjoy an experience, we might want to do it again. The driving force is born of pleasure. It may be that we enjoy being with someone and want to do more of that. It may be that we enjoy playing a sport—it gives us pleasure. You get the idea; it is all about wanting more pleasure.

On the other hand, gluttony is all about not having enough. Imagine this scenario. Three people are at a table and a pizza is ordered to share. Each person takes a slice and one slice remains. Two of the three enjoy eating their slice whilst having a conversation in between bites. The third scoffs the food down fast enough to be able to beat the others to grab the last slice of pizza.

Gluttony is born of fear. The fear is that there is not enough to go round and, therefore, what is available must be grabbed fast, just in case someone else gets it first. It tends to be concealed well by some who, with time, become experts at positioning themselves to take advantage of second helpings and leftovers.

Fear and greed are driving forces behind our actions. We tend to be going towards something we want because it is pleasurable and brings us joy or moving away from something to avoid discomfort and fear.

Regrettably, the majority of decisions we make are born of fear. Something that may help is grasping that the core of any decision is determined by the driving force behind it.

For example, a woman goes to the doctor to find out what is preventing her from having a baby. The doctor suggests that the woman is 30 percent above her maximum body weight and suggests that unless she reduces her weight, she is unlikely to get pregnant.

On hearing this, she starts a rigorous regime of weight loss, measuring everything and obsessively counting calories. This may result in a fear of getting onto the scales and worrying that she is not shedding the excess quickly enough; she may even further cut her food intake.

There are two different ways of perceiving the doctor's prognosis. On one hand is the fear that she may not be able to procreate unless she loses weight, and so she attempts to force her body to make a dramatic and quite a challenging change.

On the other hand, this situation may be perceived very differently. The doctor's advice could be seen as a great result, in that she has found a solution to her inability to conceive and she will be able to increase her agility and mobility in the process.

The former reaction is fear driven, whilst the latter is all about getting more out of life. It is all about how we choose to perceive the situation. If we see it as something constructive that we want, then it is possible to make a pleasure-based decision.

The Power of the Mind

The mind is the principle orchestrator of the events in our lives. Equipped with powerful abilities, it handles our choices and creates automated responses to minimize risk and energy.

Our mind plays a significant part in managing not only our daily activities but also our functional needs. In essence, it is a self-organizing, self-actualizing, and pattern-making mechanism. What this means is that it organizes information (in formation) so as to enable us to act and react in the fulfillment of our needs and wants.

It is much like a "blank slate," to use a Stephen Pinker term; it has little preconceived idea of what to expect and what to do with what happens. What this means to us is that the mind needs to collate information through its senses and give meaning to them in a way that allows us to relate to the world around us.

The information received is stored in such a way that it forms patterns on condition that they are stable and functional. We learn from whatever is going on around us. This can be seen in young children who want to know everything. "Why" is a very popular word with children, certainly from the age of two onwards. The more we know, the less likely the chances of being caught out, and the safer we feel.

Our Mind Needs Patterns

Uncertainty is to be avoided at all costs, as far as the mind is concerned. When it comes to our survival, our ability to nourish our body is perhaps the most important first rule for survival.

Understand that the mind creates patterns for us to follow, like roadways that take us places. Patterns are pre-programmed actions that we do not have to think about. Just to demonstrate this, imagine that each morning we put on nine pieces of clothing. If we did not have a pattern to follow and had to learn each morning how to get dressed, it could take up to 362 tries before we got it right.

It seems that without our mind having this ability, we would have perished off the face of the planet. Fortunately, this ability has allowed us to learn from our predecessors and adapt to the ever-changing demands of the world that we live in and the society that we cohabit.

The way we shop, the tastes we acquire, the volume we consume, the brands we choose, etc., are all revelations of patterns that preexist in our psyche. We think we have choice when in fact we have conditional choice. Once we have started down a path, we tend not to know that we can stop and go back or do something different. We might even say to ourselves that we could change our minds, yet find ourselves choosing to do what we have already chosen.

It would be impossible for us to stay constantly aware of everything in our lives. Yet awareness is one the essential ingredients to changing anything in our lives. If we are not aware of something, then it is not in our mind and therefore it does not exist. Additionally, where the mind has accepted a situation as normal, it is because it has become an instinctive response; it is, in other words, thoughtless.

Awareness requires focused concentration.

The mind is not aware of what it is not focused on. If we are eating something on the fly whilst having a conversation on the telephone, playing a video game, or watching a film, we are not always conscious of what we are doing.

Our Emotional States

The way the mind responds to emotional information is by sending a signal to our consciousness and, at the same time, a separate signal to a part of the brain called the amygdala. The journey to the amygdala is faster and, consequently, we react emotionally much faster than we do consciously.

What this means to us is that if we are experiencing something emotionally, we react instinctively. Conscious reasoning and logical reactions take longer to occur. It is no wonder, then, that we are trapped by the efficiency of our unconscious reactions to stressful situations.

To be in control of our weight requires that we plan for many eventualities, occasionally though we may react in a destructive way to stressful situations. Our reaction time is critical if we are not to be manipulated by our emotions. Our reaction to stress needs to be better managed.

Stress

It is prudent to work on the factors that create stress as well as to be better informed about what we are eating and the effect that food is having on us.

Stress comes about as a result of not having sufficient resources to cope with the demands that we have invited or have had placed upon us. Suffice it to say that when our body is left to cope with persistent stress, something that it was never designed to do, we are left exhausted and either break down or burn out. Both states are damaging to our psyche and body.

Habits

Habits are formed over years, months, weeks, days, and even hours. They tend to be things that occur through repetition. We become used to picking up the phone when it rings; we do not have to think, "What is that sound?" We automatically just step into a routine. Habits are routines that we follow without thought.

Routines are essential for our survival. We need them to make our life more manageable and more certain. Whilst engaging with any routine, we can still be aware of other things. When we are cooking up the usual Tuesday night dinner or when we go to our favorite restaurant and order our usual platter, we follow a routine. As we tie our shoes, we follow a routine.

Things once learned become automated. When we consider just how much automation occurs in our everyday life, it is no wonder that it is hard to change. Just moving the cupboards around and having the tea and coffee in a different place may cause frustration.

To change our behavior, we need to change our habits. This first requires that we become aware of the habit itself, and then seek to block its path. Consider going to the supermarket; ponder just how much of that process is automated. We might use a list of items or go by memory. The probability is that you shop for the same items week in, week out.

We have a program running that tells us what to replace in our home. We rarely challenge it; we just go through the process, get to the checkout, and off to our home. We unpack the shopping and carry on as usual. Little if any thought goes towards this process.

What needs to happen, if we want things to be different, is to change our habit to one that is in keeping with the experience we want to have in our lives. If that experience is to feel physically lighter, more agile, and have more energy, then the habits we have developed over time need to change.

It is relatively simple in theory to have change; in practice it is a different matter. There is a natural resistance to the changing of any pattern. It does help if we have grown up to be willful and strong headed when it is used to our greater good.

If we carry on doing what we have always done, it would be madness to expect things to be different. By removing temptation from a weak will, we can go a long way to making change happen. It cannot be done halfheartedly. We must plan for one outcome, and that needs to be success.

Planning is an important part of the change process in any area of life. To break habits requires a great deal of planning and organizing.

Having said this, do not underestimate the ability for our mind to resist changing anything that it has learned to live with. Therefore, habits need to be considered as the enemy of change.

Compulsions

If habits are things we just do, compulsions are things we have to do. They are not as easy to deal with as habits, though there is a way if our will is determined to change our weight.

Compulsions are deeper; their roots are buried in our psyche. "I have to eat the other bar of chocolate because otherwise there are an odd number of bars left in the pack." Compulsions can vary from one person to another in their expression, yet they serve a similar purpose. The relief of anxiety caused by a stressful situation can be evidenced in some people with compulsive behaviors.

If you find yourself eating compulsively or behaving in ways that distress you, we would suggest that a visit to your physician for an assessment might well be of benefit.

Obsessive behaviors tend to be characterized by individuals who cannot *not* perform an act. This can cause deep frustration for the individual and also for his or her loved ones. It is by no means limited to checking locks and light switches; it can extend to a regime that includes foods and beverages.

There is a similarity between addiction and compulsion. We have to have this or that. Chocolate addicts will recognize this type of compulsion. We visit a shop and find it almost impossible to leave the counter without picking up the chocolate bar.

Once more, if you find yourself in that situation, it would be prudent to seek professional assistance from a physician or specialist. Only by dealing with the cause of the anxiety that causes the behavior can you focus on making changes through weight loss.

CB

IN CONCLUSION:

- Be aware of the relationship you have with food and eating—watch out for psychological triggers that may cause you to overeat unhealthy foods. Explore your presuppositions and challenge where they no longer serve your best interest.

- Our mind is averse to change and will do what it can to maintain its present course. Only you can make change happen. Remember that you can't make change happen by just saying what you are going to do. Change happens only when you make it happen in reality.

- Be aware of your habits and compulsions relating to food.

Chapter 6.
Your Best Body Within

IN A NUTSHELL:

- Waking up to the reality of their current size and weight can be a shock for some people. For some, this shock spurs them into action; for others, they manage to bury the reality and carry on as usual.

- Some give up on their goal of losing weight because they've had unsuccessful attempts in the past using very low-calorie diets or complex, convoluted diet systems.

- Successful weight loss will require an initial investment in terms of time, planning, and determination. We will need to be focused and set realistic goals. Weight loss takes time and patience.

- Be aware that some of the people in your life may not want to see you successfully change and may even look to sabotage your progress. Also be aware of self-sabotage, where those little "nibbles" and "treats" may undermine your progress; keep a food diary initially.

- Avoid comparing yourself with others; focus on your own progress and actualizing your best shape. Observe your beliefs about your size, weight, shape, and eating habits, and challenge these where necessary.

- There are certain varying body type characteristics and genes that control, to a degree, how lean an individual can be. This is a reason that comparing yourself with others is usually unproductive and often frustrating.

- No matter what your current size, eating healthily over the long term will optimize *your* body shape. You will become the best physical version of yourself that you can be. Being in the best shape you can be has many advantages, including being able to look after yourself well into your golden years.

❀

It can be scary to discover that you do not look as you had hoped you looked. It's a sudden realization that the person you thought you were is not the person you really are.

That image of yourself is not what you had perpetuated in your mind. In fact, the reality could even be an image that may disgust you. Yet somehow, many people need to find a way to conceal what their eyes witnessed, sufficiently to be able to carry on their everyday life. Self-deception is not an easy thing at times like these.

People need to find ways to cope with their brief encounter with their real physical self. It is not easy to deal with this awakening. It is not easy to go back to the illusion. Yet most people do so without too much discomfort. Justifications, excuses, comparisons, circumstances, and the like are used to quickly dissolve the horror of reality.

A client who came for some assistance said:

> I had been on a business trip with one of my partners
> to Chicago. On our arrival back in London, the
> aircraft was parked a distance from the main terminal
> with a heck of a walk to check out of immigration.
>
> Our luggage had to be picked up and carried for this
> long walk. At a certain point, I had got ahead of my
> partner and stopped to rest. As I did, I saw someone
> walking towards me, bloblike, huffing, puffing, and
> looking very distraught. Suddenly I realized that it
> was my partner, whom I had always considered
> smaller than me in size. Until that moment, I had not
> seen him as fat, just big. What I saw was a fat man
> that looked sweaty and distorted.
>
> My whole body juddered when I stopped and
> deliberately looked at my own reflection. I froze at
> the realization that I looked bigger than my partner
> did. Somehow, I had managed over many years to
> trick myself into believing that I was only a little
> overweight based on how my partner looked.
>
> It was only then that I stopped and pondered on
> what I really looked like. It seems denial of the truth
> was the trap that I had fallen into. Self-made and self-
> imposed. Without a second to waste, I started to look
> at myself differently and decided that I could not live
> with the thought that I was fat. Yes, at thirty-two

years of age, I had reached three hundred and thirty six pounds (one hundred and fifty two kilograms).

Sometimes a little self-examination might bring new perspectives that could seriously help improve the quality of our lives. Solutions are not discovered unless the problem is acknowledged.

Before you go on reading, have a good long look at your body, gently grab an area of your excess, and decide if it is something you want to accept or something you want to lose.

If the answer is to be free of the excess, then read on and discover the mechanics, the psychology, and some simple solutions that will help set you free.

If, on the other hand, you don't like it and at the same time believe that there is nothing you can do about it, having read this book, then we would strongly suggest that you truly accept your size, and move on with your life.

How Do You Stay the Size You Are?

Often we are unaware that we do have the ability to control our weight and body size to some extent. The premise is simple. Let us assume that currently we weigh two hundred pounds or ninety kilograms. Perhaps there is a fluctuation from time to time, but generally we maintain this weight.

The question to ponder on is this: how are we able to maintain this body weight and not allow it to increase to two hundred and ten pounds or ninety five kilograms? We already have a strategy to maintain our two hundred pound or ninety kilogram weight and we know (even if only subconsciously) how not to allow it to get up to two hundred and ten pounds or ninety five kilograms.

Common sense tells us that if we are able to maintain a weight, we are to a degree in control of that weight. It just so happens that we are at a weight that we are not completely comfortable with. Take a moment and consider the actions we would decide to take if one morning we woke up having gone to bed weighing two hundred pounds or ninety kilograms and the next morning we look in the mirror and discover that we have grown to three hundred pounds or one hundred and thirty six kilograms.

I know you may be thinking that this is not possible. Just stay with us, because although it is not possible overnight it certainly can be possible over a period of months. Let's stay with the possibility just for a few minutes. What are we likely to do after we have run around like a lunatic, phoned a friend or ten, and started to research on the Net what could have happened to us, what disease we may have caught?

We would probably throw out all foods that we know to be unhealthy for us, anything that would be adding to our weight. So out go the sweets, chocolates, ice cream, pastas, pizza, bread, etc.

We would probably stop alcohol, sodas, and colas and replace them with water; we would in effect start taking care of ourselves. We would be disinterested in what others are eating and only focus on ourselves with the limited resources we have.

The point is this, why wait to get to that place before we take action? It is as though for some people, only shock will drive them. The danger at that point is that it may be too late to do anything about the fat weight. It is one thing climbing a mountain when you have a small backpack and another when it is full of kaka.

THE CHALLENGES OF LOSING WEIGHT:

Perhaps you have previously had a go at losing weight and given up. It could be that you realized it was harder than you had imagined.

Sometimes we buy a piece of furniture from a catalogue and assume that the putting together is going to be a cinch. When it arrives, we find we are unable to understand the directions for self-assembly, and we give in until someone comes to fix it. We buy an electronic appliance and end up giving it to someone else because we do not really understand it. It is unlikely that we would say, "I don't get it." We might just say, "I don't use this anymore."

The difficulty, especially for people who experienced this type of failure, is that insufficient time was given to the full implications of losing weight. Why should it not be easy? Why, most everything else in our life comes easy? Doesn't it?

Have you noticed the thing that comes really easy is the advertisement selling the food that makes us fat that is so easy to get hold of!

Unfortunately, the things that matter in life are not always easy to get. Losing fat weight is one of them. Stop before you compare your body with models in advertisements, celebrities in magazines, your neighbors or friends, or even your colleague in the office; they are not you.

Some people attempt to make themselves feel better because they are smaller than the person next to them. This is a wonderfully simple way to distort reality sufficiently enough to satisfy their ego.

In any event, a real investment needs to be made in terms of time and determination. Either do this or not; the yo-yo diet is a loser's game. The stress and tension on our body are in some cases catastrophic.

Perhaps weight loss in the past was slower and took longer than we had imagined.

Imagine people getting on a train that is travelling to another city. The departure and arrival times are clearly printed on the ticket. As they check their watches, they think that they should be halfway through their journey, only to discover that the train on this occasion is only a quarter of the way there.

They complain to the conductor and rage at how terrible the service is. The conductor apologizes and says that he will report their complaint. Not satisfied at this, they tell the conductor that they are so disgusted at this that they will get off at the next station and get another train. The reasoning is simple: why should we put up with something that does not do exactly what it says on the label? To hell with them, we will wait for the one that works properly.

This philosophy is not uncommon for some who are not able to adjust their thinking so as to serve their greater good. Pride can blind us from the evidence in front of us. Common sense has left the building. We do need to pause and review our progress and accept that hurdles appearing on our journey are not a sign to quit.

It could be that there were too many stressors and distractions for us.

An often-made, simple mistake is deciding to start weight loss in the midst of major changes to our routines. We are about to change jobs or homes; we are having relationship difficulties; perhaps a loss of a loved one; there may be too many financial demands imposed upon us; there may be too many expectations levied on us.

We need to seriously consider what pressure we are under and take a stand on how we will deal with the pressures, so as to be able to calmly focus on our weight loss.

Planning, determination, and timing are important aspects of successful weight loss.

It could also be that we never challenged the evidence scientifically and therefore went for the wrong weight loss program.

Learn to challenge everything relating to food intake. Without the need to become obsessed, find time to read and research enough to gain a better understanding of your needs.

It may be that a saboteur infiltrated our program.

Remember that not everyone will necessarily enjoy your success. They may not declare any hostility, but others often fear our success, and what may happen if we accomplish our goal. It is not unlike someone who knows we are being aware about what we eat and they relish the moments when they can stuff their face in front of us.

They could perhaps be stupid, manipulative, or incapable of empathy. In any event, they may not be people we want around during our transition. Only when we have a stable and established position in relation to our dietary needs can we be indifferent to their behavior.

Self-sabotage is perhaps the real danger.

Eric Hoffer said, "We lie loudest when we lie to ourselves." He was certainly right about that. The reason is that this type of lie is unbeatable. Only we can know the truth of what we ate and what we left.

Food diaries are a must for anyone who wants to beat subconscious or even willful self-deception. We might also suggest that your whole notion of fat loss needs to be reviewed and a decision taken to be sincere in your intentions.

This type of sabotage can also be found in little habits that allow us to have nibbles here and there that undermine our efforts for temporary gratification and result in a greater degree of duress. It is like asking your dentist to pull a tooth out a little bit at a time over the next few years.

If your intention is only to begin to focus on your weight loss when you reach a certain weight or cannot fit into a certain clothes size, then it's simple. Pile on the pounds and get there sooner so you can start to act faster.

Remember to Focus on Yourself

We propose a way to measure success by simply focusing on yourself. The degree of comfort you experience being in your skin is what matters. How does it feel to be you? Don't compare yourself to pictures of others in magazines and the media that look to project an unrealistic image of humans. We are humans that share similar habits and characteristics, not minds and bodies, nor needs and wants.

Your Beliefs

We self-actualize our beliefs. Beliefs are the core of 99 percent of what happens to us. The other 1 percent is chance. Our beliefs are the patterns that we are predisposed to repeating. Beliefs are the result of evidence that supports a view that is in keeping with the existing evidence.

We amass millions of beliefs about the world and thousands about ourselves. They tend to be fixed, as if in stone and ridged. Yet mostly they are outdated and maintained through historical continuity.

Beliefs are our personal truths. In other words, they are true to us. The oddity is that the mind has an amazing ability to hold opposing views. We can believe that we are nice and kind, that we are good people, that we are gentle, attractive, and soft, that we are thoughtful and considerate to ourselves and to others.

We can also believe that we are angry and insensitive, that we are impatient and thoughtless, that we are right and the rest of the world is wrong, that we are ugly, fat, big, and unattractive. We are capable of cruelty and hostility. Two sides of the same coin. As far as our mind is concerned, both sides are true. In some instances, we switch from one to the other in milliseconds.

We can look in the mirror, do that magic wiggle and wink, and go out with a spring in our step, thinking that we look sexy and cool, that we are adorable and eye catching, that we are great, fabulous, and smart. In a blink of a thought, we can be thinking the opposite.

It is interesting that our mind can flip with such ease from one state to another. There is a raft of evidence that supports the theory that we can, with practice, change at will from one state of being to another. Exercises in the strategies section will help you with this.

Base Your Expectations in Reality

It is possible to metabolize one to two pounds or 0.5 to one kilogram of fat a week. Think how long it took you to put on weight—you didn't just wake up fat one morning. Set a realistic goal. An example of a sensible goal for someone with fourteen pounds or six kilograms of fat to lose is twelve weeks. Write down your personal goal and stick it up somewhere you will see it—the fridge door is good.

To look at other people and compare yourself with them is laced with dangers. Remember that what you focus on and direct your mind towards is, in most respects, instructing your mind to go in that direction. Stop and review your purpose in comparing yourself with others.

Some people just look and play the "her butt is bigger than mine" game, which conveniently bolsters or satisfies their ego and suggests that their own body is better. Comparisons like this are not only useless; they are also extremely dangerous.

Getting to grips with your body's shape and size has little if anything to do with someone else's body. There are so many factors involved in body types that it is completely worthless. Furthermore, it may be that you are gaining a momentary buzz in believing you are smaller than the person you are comparing yourself with, when, in fact, you are distorting what you are seeing to satisfy your need to continue doing what you are doing. This is another way of maintaining self-deception.

We are suggesting that if we perceive we are smaller than the other person, we have reached our goal and therefore our mind need do no more to make adjustments.

Weight or fat gain is a highly individual trait. Some people can put excess weight on very easily, yet for others it is hard to do, no matter how many calories they eat.

There really is a large variability between individuals due to a combination of genetic and hormonal factors. There are no two ways about it—there is no use blaming yourself and no use wishing you had another person's body or body type. We have to play the hand we have been dealt. What we have a choice in is how well we play our particular hand.

What are the reasons that there are so many different body types when we look at the wider population?

We all have individual hereditary information passed on to us from our parents in the form of genes (a gene is a unit of genetic information). There is a specific gene called the "ob gene" which dictates how much body fat we as individuals are likely to store. Some people are designed to carry more body fat than others, and this is a part of our individual genetic code. This doesn't mean that we have to be resigned to being overweight. What it does mean is we need to be realistic in our expectations of how individually we can look our best.

A simple example, to take two extremes, is that an Olympic shot-putter is never going to look like an Olympic marathon runner. This is not down to the type of physical training these two sports people undertake—it is primarily down to their body type and genetic makeup.

Focus on Being the Best *You* Can Be

Notice the physiques of a typical female Olympic shot-putter and an Olympic female marathon runner. It is a misconception to believe that their bodies are purely the result of their athletic training.

These individuals have excelled at their particular sport not because of dedication and training alone. There is a factor of much more fundamental importance to their being Olympic athletes. They started out with exceptional body types for their particular sports; the genetics they inherited dictated what they could physically excel at.

The role of our genetics is a key to setting ourselves appropriate fat loss goals that are reachable and realistic for us, just as an Olympic shot-putter is never going to be an Olympic marathon runner and vice versa.

Only a certain percentage of the population has the ability to be Kate Moss thin, and if you don't start out with the right genetic material to naturally look like that, it's never going to happen for you. You will simply be frustrating yourself and having an antagonistic relationship with who you are.

Here is another example: Kate Moss could never have a body that looks like Beyonce's, and Beyonce could never have a body that looks like Kate Moss's. No amount of sensible dieting or extreme dieting or exercise could give either woman a figure that looks like the other's. Their starting points are different. They have different body types, and if one wished to have the other's figure, that's all they would have—a wish, and then frustration that no matter what they do, they cannot look like the image they have in their mind.

Acceptance of *your* body type is a key to successful fat loss. A dress size of 0 in the United States or 4 in the United Kingdom is likely to be downright unhealthy as well as unobtainable for most women. Some women's best size possible may be 8-10 in the United States or 12-14 in the United Kingdom. It is really important to look at yourself with clarity and self-understanding of what is likely your best.

Somatotypes

Dr. William H. Sheldon developed the theory of somatotypes, describing three basic human body types: endomorph, mesomorph, and ectomorph. These are applicable to both men and women.

Endomorphs tend to have a more rounded appearance and are often susceptible to putting on excess weight. In women, their hips are often wider than their shoulders.

Mesomorphs tend to have strong, athletic builds. They can build muscle and lose weight more easily than the other somatotypes. Their shoulders are generally wider than their hips.

Ectomorphs tend to be thin, slim or even underweight. They tend to have narrow hips and shoulders. They typically have a challenge gaining weight and building muscle.

Many people do not strictly fall into one category: endomorph, mesomorph, or ectomorph. Often we tend to be a combination of two of these body types.

Now the good news is that although some of us may have genetics that make it more likely that we will store more body fat than the next person, it does not mean we have to be overly fat or unattractive.

The biological science of epigenetics has shown that diet (and other environmental factors like exercise) can effectively switch on or off certain hereditary genetic information (genes) in our personal DNA (the nucleic acid where our genetic instructions are stored). So even if your DNA at birth makes it more likely for you to store body fat, if you eat healthily and perform a sensible amount of exercise, you can manipulate your genetic information to favor being lean.

Conversely, poor nutrition will only emphasize or turn on the genes that make it more likely for you to gain weight. If you stick with eating healthily over time, your body will actually begin to favor being in a lean state. It will become more natural for you. This effect has even been shown to be passed on to offspring for up to four generations. So how you look after yourself can potentially impact in a very beneficial way on your children and further down the family line.[1]

Naturally skinny people are not necessarily healthy either. If they eat unhealthy food over the long term, they may not look outwardly fat thanks to their genetics, but they can build up unhealthy and potentially dangerous amounts of visceral fat around their internal organs. They are often just as much at risk from many of the diet-related illnesses associated with metabolic syndrome as those who store body fat more easily.

Knowing your body type and shape can empower you and enable you to set realistic, obtainable goals for yourself. Once we have accepted the benefits and challenges of the body we are born with, we can stop comparing ourselves to others and focus on becoming the best *we* can be.

As We Age, Size Still Matters

Recently we have been engaged in helping a friend aid her parents with a misadventure.

Our friend's mother fell badly when rising from her chair. She fainted, and the next thing she knew she was flat on her face and looked like she had been in a knockout boxing competition. When we arrived, we called the ambulance, and they decided to take her to a local hospital.

From a seated position, they moved her into a chair and wheeled her out and into the ambulance. The process was quite challenging for the two ambulance men even though she was able to stand up on her own.

A few weeks later and we got a phone call to say that she had fallen again, this time down the stairs and over the banister. We discovered afterward that she broke her arm, wrist, finger, and three ribs. Needless to say, the ambulance was called and arrived while we were there. She was lying on the floor, reeling in agony, unable to communicate coherently.

Suffice it to say the emergency response unit and ambulance men decided to take her to hospital again. She looked like she had put on a few more pounds in the intervening weeks. When it came to lifting her from the floor into the chair, it was like a scene from a dark film.

It took three people to lift her. It was quite an undignified event that is best forgotten. There is an important message here for those who seek value in disposing of unnecessary and excess weight. Not being able to hold your own weight has some massive disadvantages. It is worth considering that with age comes less movement and agility.

The point being that when evaluating the value of not carrying too much fat, we need to consider benefits that may not be apparent and appreciated until much later on in life.

&

In conclusion:

- Base your expectations in reality. Set yourself realistic goals—aim for one to two pounds or 0.5 to one kilogram of fat loss per week. There is no need and no point in making comparisons with others; instead, keep track of your physical condition and chart your progress caringly.

- Look out for those people who seek to demoralize and disempower you. They may come appearing to care whilst in reality they have a hidden agenda. Avoid the blame game and accept that you and only you are in control of what you put in your mouth.

- Where no goal has been set, the mind will keep doing what it has always done, by default. Setting and keeping a goal in mind instructs the mind as to where you are heading. Keep focused, keep realistic expectations, and relentlessly maintain your desire for a healthier shape and size.

- Planning, determination, and timing are important aspects of successful weight loss.

Chapter 7.
Excess Fat—What Winners Lose

IN A NUTSHELL:

- Weighing scales don't tell the full picture—we won't know whether weight lost or gained comes from water, muscle, or fat. Obsessive weighing can undermine our good intentions.

- If the scale shows no weight loss, we may get angry. Yet our weight may have stayed the same due to an increase in muscle tissue at the same time as fat loss. The constant use of weighing scales only erodes your personal power and suggests doubt in your abilities to accomplish your goal.

- If you are going to use scales, only do so once a week, at the same time, on the same day. If one week's readings don't show improvement, stay calm—only if a trend happens for two or three weeks in a row will you need to reassess your diet.

- Fluid retention can fluctuate by as much as five pounds or two kilograms in a single day for some people. This is true particularly for women during their monthly cycle.

- If you slip up on your diet or have a "cheat" day, don't be surprised if your scale weight jumps up. Most of this increase will be water rather than fat—so long as it is only a short-term slip up. Obviously fat will accumulate again if you continually eat poorly.

Ↄ

The Weigh-In

Here's how fat loss occurs: when the body's sources of glycogen are somewhat exhausted, we begin to use our own fat stores for energy (lipolysis). Our stored fat cells are broken down into glycerol and fatty acids, which are used to make energy. We can then use this energy for our everyday needs and our fat weight reduces.

Using scales to monitor weight loss may not be the best solution for most people. Size and shape matter more. The scales for some people can become an obsessive pastime. In fact, we can become so focused on the weight that we are in danger of developing an angry relationship with the scales.

The experience that we have is what matters. If the relationship with the scales becomes the most important aspect of our weight loss, then you can imagine what is not getting our attention. We may approach our nutritional needs with an attitude that is likely to result in failure.

When the scales become all that matters, the battle is lost. There are a few exceptions to the rule; some people may have an obsessive nature, which requires them to fixate on the scales and drive themselves until they reach "that weight." They tend to be driven by an "I will show you attitude," and, come hell or high water, they will.

For most others it seems that the scales simply evidence their inability to accomplish a set weight. For such people it is more than likely that what they will go on to accomplish is a lifelong relationship with the scales that results in frustration and disappointment.

Scales can be useful things, as are mirrors, and they are there to serve a purpose. They will not correct the situation, only highlight what is. The danger is that we can keep focused on the negative for so long that we are self-programming a weight or size that we do not want to be, over and over again.

If the scales work for you and you have noticed the benefit, then carry on using them. If, though, you notice that the scale weighing is creating a negative experience, such as disappointment or despair, then get off until your attitude can be changed to one that is in keeping with your best interests.

When reducing our weight, it is important to keep in mind the difference between general weight loss and fat loss, because they are not the same. Weight loss is all encompassing; it can be due to a reduction in fat, muscle, and fluid (water) combined.

We certainly do not want to lose muscle whilst dieting, as this will reduce our metabolic rate—the number of calories our bodies use to sustain ourselves. If we lose muscle, it will be harder to lose more body fat and far easier to put more fat on in the future because of our reduced metabolic rate.

This is the reason that weighing ourselves on scales is the least preferred method of gauging fat loss—because we don't know what we are losing, whether it is fat, muscle, or fluid. In addition, we could step on the scale and note that our weight has stayed the same or increased, and this may cause us to become disheartened, believing that our efforts over the previous week or two have been to no avail, when this may not be the case at all.

We may have lost two pounds or one kilogram of fat, gained a pound or 0.5 kilogram of muscle, and our fluid levels may happen to be up by a pound or 0.5 kilogram in weight on the day/time that we weigh ourselves. In this scenario, our scale weight remains the same as two weeks ago, yet actually there has been fat loss, which is beneficial, and there has been muscle gain, which is healthy.

A further factor to bear in mind with weighing yourself on scales is that water retained in the body may fluctuate over the course of a day by several pounds or kilograms. This alone can throw off the accuracy of any scale reading for someone focused on losing *fat*.

How to Measure Your Progress

So what is the most appropriate way to measure our progress whilst on a fat reduction diet? Well, the most accurate scientific methods are hydrostatic body composition tests or body caliper measurements.

The first is not practical or affordable for most people. The caliper tests can be quite accurate, but for greatest accuracy, you will need to find a professional to take your measurements. There are some self-testing calipers available that can get reasonably accurate results depending on your skill at taking the readings yourself.

What about the scales which claim to measure body fat? These can be very inaccurate and deceptive. The problem lies in all the different algorithms and averages these scales use as well as skin conductivity issues. We would not recommend relying on these at all.

Ultimately, all the gadgets that are manufactured and sold claiming to accurately measure your body fat levels are at best occasionally accurate and many times not. The real issue with this is the frustration and needless questioning of your success in terms of fat loss.

The best way to assess your fat loss is noticing the way your clothes fit, looking at photos of your body, and, if you feel the need to be a little more scientific, then taking tape measurements of your waist, hips, thighs, and arms with a tailor's-style tape measure (one that will not stretch or warp over time). This is by far the best method we can use to monitor our progress.

If you do decide to use the tape measure, make sure you always measure in exactly the same spots for accuracy, and only measure yourself every two to four weeks. Avoid getting obsessed about it.

Women need to avoid taking measurements on the days immediately before, during, and after their monthly cycle, as the readings will be inaccurate due to retention of fluids. In fact, for women we would recommend measuring just once a month, as far away from ovulation as possible.

Another point important for both men and women is not to take any measurements in the hours after any kind of exercise. In the case of high-intensity strength training, performed once a week as detailed in chapter 12, take measurements before your workout, on the day of your workout (this would obviously be six days after your last workout).

Always check the way your clothes fit or take your measurements at the same time of day—ideally, if you can, first thing in the morning, soon after you've risen from bed.

Fluid retention affects women in particular, but also men, and body weight can fluctuate by five pounds (two kilograms) or more in a single day for some people. This is why it is important to view your body shape and size over the long term and look for long-term patterns, rather than the error many overzealous dieters make of weighing themselves every day. They end up getting frustrated by what is actually perfectly normal fluctuation in overall bodyweight and nothing at all to do with fat gain.

It is the short-term view that is so often damaging to people's success. Think long term; you didn't put on all your excess fat overnight, and to believe that you can lose it overnight is undermining your success.

You don't wake up one morning suddenly fat, and you don't wake up the next morning suddenly thin either. Focus on making the right choices day by day as best you can, and every two months you will lose around a stone (sometimes for some people more, sometimes for some people a little less) if you have that much weight to lose. In time, you will have the best body weight you can achieve.

I thought you could only lose around one to two pounds or 0.5 to one kilogram of fat a week, but I've only just started your diet and I've lost way more than that in my first couple of weeks! What's happening?

Whilst it is accurate that the human body can typically only metabolize or "burn off" roughly one to two pounds or 0.5 to one kilogram of actual fat in a week, when you begin our way of eating, you will lose excess and unnecessarily retained water weight in the first few weeks of changing your diet.

Some people may lose three to four pounds or two kilograms of body weight per week for the first few weeks; for others, particularly those who carry a lot of excess body weight or those who are obese, weight loss could be as high as ten pounds or five kilograms per week for the first few weeks. Of this weight lost, it is likely that two pounds or one kilogram will have been fat and the rest will be from water.

This same situation is true of many diets—and it largely reflects on the reduction in refined carbohydrate intake, no matter what type of diet a person is on; you may have noticed this for yourself in the past.

What causes this water retention in the first place? Eating a diet that contains grains, sugars, and hydrogenated fats causes unhealthy water retention. This water is retained in and between the cells throughout our body—we are actually in a state of systemic inflammation. This can put unnecessary pressure on our heart and cardiovascular systems.

This is how so many fad diets can claim "Lose twenty pounds in two weeks." It may be a true statement, but it is certainly misleading to some degree (because it is not twenty pounds of fat the person will have lost), and this will cause mental anguish for the dieter if she believes she will continue to lose weight at that rate.

Once the body has brought its water levels down to natural healthy levels in the first few weeks of a diet, that's it; any future water loss will be minimal or nonexistent, and from then on, a person eating a healthy weight loss diet will be losing about one to two pounds or 0.5 to one kilogram a week.

It is very important to understand that the amount of weight lost during the first two to four weeks of a diet is exceptional. It does not reflect the norm from the four-week point on, unless of course a person slips up, retains more water again, then gets back on track, and then loses that water.

Any time a person slips up on his or her diet and, say over the course of a weekend, consumes some products containing grains, sugars, or hydrogenated fats again, there is likely to be a disproportionate gain in weight.

Some of this weight gain may be fat, but much is from the return of water retention. This is why a little slipup can seem such a massive issue for dieters that don't know this. It seems like one step forward and two steps back—as if one or two little slipups cause an unfair amount of weight to be put back on. It is at this point some people consider giving up their diet because "it doesn't work for me" or "it's too hard."

It is important to remember that if you do slip up, that newly regained weight that is causing a four pounds or two kilograms increase on the scales over the course of a single weekend is mostly water retention—and it will come off very quickly as soon as you start eating right again.

Now this is not an excuse to allow you to keep going off the rails because "it doesn't matter, it's only water weight." That attitude too will undo any long-term fat loss success. However, it is important information to know and will allow you to have realistic expectations for long-term fat loss.

So enjoy those first few weeks where you may lose startling amounts of weight, then remember to focus on and congratulate yourself for the one or two pounds or 0.5 to one kilogram a week of actual fat you will be losing until you achieve your ideal body weight.

છ

IN CONCLUSION:

- Think of long-term trends, not short-term readings—losing fourteen pounds or six kilograms in two months is good going. Even if you lose more scale weight, it is likely you will have only lost around one to two pounds or 0.5 to one kilogram of actual fat in a week. So look at your objective as long term for a long-lasting result.

- By avoiding the constant weighing and measuring, you are in effect increasing your self-belief. You will, through your actions, teach your mind that you are expecting change at the right pace and the right time, based on your new eating regime. There are many hurdles to overcome, so it does not help adding unnecessary and worthless pressure.

Chapter 8.
Powerful Planning for Success

IN A NUTSHELL:

- Plan ahead and decide a realistic weight or size you want to achieve. By learning to balance the dreamer, the pragmatist, and the critic inside yourself, you are likely to experience a newfound determination. It will also help you to establish emotional balance within your mind and body.

- Affirmations and positive self-talk can be beneficial, but they can also be harmful if not structured in a realistic way. Affirmations must contain an element of truth pertinent to you, not just wishful thinking.

- Learn what your personal anchors and triggers are with regard to your eating patterns; focus on altering the negative ones. Anchors are on the air, on billboards, in shop windows, etc. Be aware that marketers and advertisers are vying for your attention; they will make you plenty of "irresistible" offers. Resist this buy-in loop if the product on offer is not in your best interests.

- There are some specific questions in this chapter that will enable you to set an effective plan to reach your weight loss objectives. Answering these questions will help to foster successful change.

- For some people a "Just do it!" attitude is essential for success, like a horse with blinkers; their line of vision is focused only on winning the race.

- Avoid judging both yourself and others. Keep in mind that all judgment is self-judgment. What you say of and to others, you also apply to yourself. Focus on your strengths, support yourself, and show genuine care for yourself through this process. By avoiding playing the victim, "poor me," or "it's not fair" games, you will further develop your self-esteem and self-worth.

- Be aware that we can sometimes distort, delete, and generalize information to suit existing patterns in our minds. When we are looking to make changes, we need to ensure clarity in our thinking and understanding.

- Appreciate that of the words we use, some can be damaging to our mind-set and actions. These include "don't," "ought," "should," "must," "but," "try," "wish," and "hope." Also learn to say, "Thank you…no," when loved ones and friends suggest eating something or offer a gift of something you know will undo your weight loss.

- You will need to choose to change some of your nutritional habits if you are going to attain the goal of weight loss. Confident decisions and actions combined with correct persistence are essential.

- Keep a food diary at least for your first two to three weeks to ensure you are focused on what you eat.

ଔ

The Dreamer, the Pragmatist, and the Critic

Perhaps the most important first step in beginning a weight loss program is the decision to start and achieve a defined weight/size target. Here we are not talking about just starting a diet and seeing how it turns out; rather, this is a thought-through and planned approach to reducing the fat quantity that our body carries.

At the start of most successful accomplishments is a plan. Not just any plan; a plan that can be perceived as realistic and attainable. A plan that will fulfill most of our needs and wants.

It is interesting when we explore the internal dialogue that often ensues when starting a project such as a weight/fat loss program. There is a tendency to experience conflicting internal messages.

There is a wonderful action process that the late Walt Disney used to keep his people alert to their progress. Let's suppose that you have a dream of being a healthy, fit, energetic, and positive person. Perhaps *the dreamer* in you starts to imagine how you could become the kind of person you want to be and the way you want to represent yourself in your world.

As you enjoy the thought of starting such a plan, another part of your mind steps in. You start to think about how you could bring about such a dream. The thoughts start to come together: plans for cutting down on unhealthy foods, perhaps taking your own lunch into work and even beginning an exercise program.

The pragmatist practical side of your mind starts to work out where to get good food from, perhaps remembering that you have an old lunch box that would do the job, and even coming up with some lunch and dinner ideas that would work well.

All is going well until *the critic* steps in and begins to demolish the idea. Thoughts of past failures challenge the idea that you could ever succeed at anything. The hassle and time all this will take. That you are incapable of maintaining such a plan, that you are weak willed, and it will all just end in tears and disappointment. Perhaps that you have had many of these crazy ideas in the past and you do not have what it takes.

There is enough negativity for the pragmatist to doubt that this is possible, and the dream is soon crushed. A feeling of despair emerges and you suddenly find yourself disheartened and beaten by the whole idea. The dream is lost, and whatever you perceived as possible is dismissed and considered as yet another failure.

What occurred here is relatively common for some who seem never to get off the starting blocks. Even if you were to have made a start at the first hurdle and then you trip, a torrent of "You see? You can't do this—in fact, you might as well give up now" thoughts emerge. Stop and listen to the level of criticism. Is it justified?

It might be understandable if your dream was to lose two stones in a month and become fit by the end of the week. Perhaps your dream demands that you begin with changing your diet overnight and expecting to find all-natural products and start first thing in the morning. Stop and evaluate your resources and capabilities carefully. Be realistic. Plan for success.

It may be that you are stuck without a dream and are simply wishful thinking. Simply wishing that things could be different without having an idea of what that difference looks like is highly unlikely to bring about anything but frustration.

In essence, there are three elements that need to be congruent and configured for success. There is a part of us that needs to have imagined a different way of being. Then there is a part of us that needs to have the necessary resources to be able to deliver the idea into reality. Finally, there needs to be a part of us that acts as gatekeeper to our resources and ensures that we have made the steps manageable.

Now if, in the past, we have started projects that have resulted in failure, it is likely that our mind will want to stop that from happening again. It may be that we have overestimated our resources, and when we get down to focusing on the project, we find that we run out of steam before we even get started. It is understandable to experience an internal resistance. The critic may have a point. Some crazy "miracle diet" may well be extremely damaging to our organism.

On the other hand, if we sit about doing nothing but experience discomfort, it is understandable that we will experience internal frustration and discontent with our life. Perhaps resentment starts to set in, and things just seem to go from bad to worse.

There needs to be an acceptance to the dream possibility. There needs to be an accurate evaluation of current and available resources, and there needs to be realistic expectations if we are to proceed with confidence. When setting out your objectives, ensure that the dream is realistic, check to be sure that what you seek is attainable, then validate that it is not going to be met with predictable failure.

The dreamer in you needs to create a dream that the pragmatist in you can deliver and that the critic in you can support as much as possible. When all three parts are working together and you have harmony, then you will have increased the chances of the project succeeding immeasurably.

A successful outcome depends on balancing your needs with your resources, then having the determination to act with purpose. It may be that in the past, you have made several attempts to make a difference to your shape and size and had no success.

How Our Past Eating Patterns Have Taken Root...and Beginning the Process of Change

There tends to be so much energy given to finding something that is going to magic away the excess weight. Somehow, by taking a couple of pills or eating a "super berry" or two, it will all be better.

The endless onslaught of ever-changing nutritional information overload further adds to the confusion and desperation that invites failure to our struggle to regain our body.

Much can be achieved by understanding how the mind works. It is without doubt the most important organ in helping to manifest your desired outcome. The mind is in many ways similar to the conductor of an orchestra.

If the relationship between ourselves and our orchestra is in discord, the likelihood is that we are going to be hostage to our cravings. Also, if we are not attentive to our needs, we are likely to experience discontent.

Equally, we need to challenge until we have understood the score created by the composer. During our developmental period, our carers feed us. We are told what is good and what is not. We are told and, more importantly, shown through others' actions how to be in the future. The composers of our future behaviors, in particular regarding our health and nutrition, did what they believed was best for us, based on the resources they had at the time.

Living in our skin may require a review of our mental attitude in respect of what we have accepted as being right for us; time to look at the composition we are asking our orchestra to perform, perhaps rewrite it, add a new movement, or even change and play a new melody.

We are handed down information without necessarily considering our operating system. It is a bit like someone giving you a DOS disk to run on your Mac system, or worse, as is often the case, the program has a virus. Because mostly we trust the source of that information—after all, why wouldn't we—we accept it without challenge.

Once the information is in place, our role is virtually predetermined by that same information. Here is where our mind's unique ability to form patterns comes into play. The information becomes what we know to be reality: our personal truth.

Our mind has a four-stage learning process, and it does not know what it does not know. So as you read through this book, there are going to be many moments when you may think, "OMG, I didn't know that they do that with our food."

Now we have become aware; we are aware that we are unaware of certain facts about the foods we are consuming. We have become conscious of our ignorance and the games played at our expense. We now need to find a solution to the eating habits that are causing us year on year to increase our body fat and, consequently, our size.

Now that we are conscious of what is going on, we are in the third phase of our thinking. We are starting to master our choices and are conscious of what we are doing, slow though it may be. The better we are at developing habits, the more confidence we will have in our mind's abilities in the future to keep us safe.

Having developed new behaviors in the way we choose to eat, and the habits having taken root—in other words, we no longer think about behaving with a high degree of self-preservation when it comes to our choice of foods—we step into the fourth phase of the mind's learning process. We become unconscious of selecting and eating well. It no longer consumes us; we just get on with the pleasure of living.

Let's clarify the reasoning behind this and the importance of starting slow. We have become great at eating junk; we can name just about every *"fast-fattening takeout"* in our neighborhood. We can even guarantee that when we are away, we will be able to find its accomplices in just about any town or city.

The codependent relationship we have with *fast-fattening* food chains and products needs to be seriously examined if we are ever to change our shape to the one that makes us feel good inside and out. To do this initially requires a high degree of awareness; this uses energy and will test our patience. By becoming aware, we have found half the solution; the other half is finding an alternative to those foods and deliberately sticking to our new prolife choices.

The idea of just popping down to the supermarket, walking down the same aisles, picking the same products, and continuing as we always have needs to be curtailed. In order to do this we will initially need to allow more time to do our shopping.

We might suggest that you change where you shop to get a new perspective or walk through the supermarket in the opposite direction to that you used to go. Certain aisles will require a wide berth; they are just *"fattening traps."* Remember, a supermarket does nothing for convenience and everything to maximize its profits.

Getting back our power requires diligence and persistence. It requires that we are aware of what we are eating and the effects that pseudo-products are having on our system.

In an ideal situation, we would stop, look at what we have become addicted to, recognize the benefits of not eating processed, sugar-disguised, valueless foods and drinks, and get ourselves back to preparing our own meals wherever possible. At the same time, we need to accept that the correct weight reduction needs to be gradual and controlled. About one to two pounds or 0.5 to one kilogram in a week is great, and if it does not sound enough, just look at the difference after three months.

To succeed at weight loss, you will need to think of the long game. It's not about winning the solitary point; it's all about winning the game. The game of life is a serious business, and, as best we can, we need to eat right for our body's well-being.

Be Aware of Anchors and Triggers

Anchors are ways of securing an object like a ship or a balloon so that it does not leave a specific location. Triggers are tipping points that change something at a given time in ways that have been predetermined.

Anchoring, in neurolinguistics, is a process by which a stimulus from an internal or external source causes an automatic change in a person's behavior. Triggers are the response to the anchor, which may have been programmed at any time in our lives from birth onward.

We are surrounded by anchors and triggers; the doorbell goes and we start heading towards the entrance to see who is there. Our life is laced with triggers that go off mostly unconsciously. Some may remember the sound of the ice cream truck heading our way, playing the familiar tune, and the children all asking for some money to get an ice cream cone.

We are surrounded by stimulants that trigger emotional reactions, expressed through needs. When entering a bakery, the smells get us immediately. They trigger a desire for fresh baked bread, and we sense a compelling feeling to buy, buy, buy.

There are probably numerous daily activities that we are programmed to complete. The greeting smiles of a sales assistant put us into a responsive mood to purchase. The big clownlike character who appears to be friendly to children encourages the idea of fun and safety. These are all anchors that stimulate a response. Where that response has become anchored to an action, the deal is done. We no longer think, we just act.

To minimize the effects of the programming that has been instilled in us is by no means easy. To break these anchors, we need to be aware of them in the first place. To be aware, we need to be conscious of our behavior and challenge through reasoning the need to act without first thinking about our actions.

Let's say we are aware of a person giving us a coupon with a special offer at the nearby takeaway. Stop, think, before you act. What is his or her intention and why? We would suggest that your best interest is not at the core of his or her action.

In the same way, at the supermarket, there are endless free samples being given away. The tendency is to purchase what we have been stimulated to buy. The taste of that free sample triggers our juices, and we start to develop a desire. Combine this with the law of reciprocity, and we begin to be drawn into buying something that, had it not been suggested to us, we would never have even thought about.

Challenge everything you have accepted as being good, and review your attitude to one that best fits your needs.

The Buy-In Loop

There is a tendency for us to get caught up in a virtual buy-in loop. The buy-in is subtle yet profoundly powerful.

Our mind requires validation in terms of what to do and what not to do. Have you ever found yourself wanting something that you believe you should not have at some level? Perhaps it is something that you do not need; you simply want it and it has your attention.

You may notice that the idea seems to come from somewhere. It may be that you see someone walking in a special sort of boot. It's unusual, and it seems to have sheepskin lining. You continue with your day only to notice that another person is also wearing the same style boot.

A day or so later, you notice that others are wearing them. In fact, you start to look out for people to see if they have them on. It seems that you just notice them and all other boots stop existing. It's as if you are looking out for them. You may even get a little buzz when you notice them on someone.

You go to a shop that sells those boots and start to examine a pair. You notice that the price is high, but you start to justify it. They come from Australia, they are real sheepskin, they are unlike anything else, they are soft, etc. The point is to justify to yourself whilst reaching for the plastic card and purchasing them.

As soon as you have them, you begin to wear them, and each time you see someone wearing them, on some level you feel good. You feel good probably because you believe you made the right decision to buy them. After all, other people would not buy them if they were not worth the money. They certainly would not wear them if they did not look cool.

The feeling of having made the right decision is based on other people's choices. You may have seen someone looking good in those boots. You want to look good so 1 + 1 = 2. Buy the boots and look good.

When someone says they think that they are rather expensive, you bring on the defense. You talk about the quality of the boot and the manufacturing process, you talk about others who are wearing them (actresses, models, etc.) and that they are organic, natural, humane, ecological, comfortable, and so on.

This is how most of us fall into the trap. If you looked around and examined the things that you have around you and explored how you got to choose them, you may be surprised at how influenced you have been by magazines, posters and billboards, radio, even the charming little jingles that contain a message for a product.

Imagine you are in a supermarket; you are doing your thing and notice someone go to a shelf and pick up several packets of some-food-item. Soon after another person comes and does the same thing. As you walk along you notice that some have them in their basket. Your curiosity is now likely to be ignited, and you are likely to want to know what the attraction is. As soon as your attention is drawn toward something, you are at risk.

Stop, think, and act in accordance with your best interests.

Your attention is a commodity that everyone is desperately vying to get. It is worth a great deal of money. Put simply, if someone has your attention, then there is a strong possibility that he or she can sell you something.

To put it into context, there are companies that will pay your flight and hotel bill for a weekend away. There is just one condition that needs to be met. You need to attend a seminar for four hours while you are staying at the hotel. Failing to do so results in you having to pay the expenses of the trip yourself.

It is obvious that they are not going to pay to have a planeload of people come to a hotel unless there is something in it for them. The objective is to have your undivided attention so that they can then use the power of suggestion, the group-thinking phenomenon, and the law of reciprocation, amongst many tactics, to get you to sign up and buy a week or two of a shared ownership property.

Your attention is very valuable and needs to be treated with a great regard. It is as valuable as your money, your time, your health. They are all connected, and you are heading where your attention is drawn. Be selective and consider what is in your best interest.

Nowadays this has been fully exploited on the Internet by organizations that give many free things so that you can stay on their page, where you will be offered lots of "based on your last purchase, we think this might interest you," or "other people who bought this also bought...." You get the gist. Your attention is of great value.

You need to protect your mind from wandering into the corporate matrix. Once you are in, you will be milked daily until you are done. Getting out is not as easy as we would like it to be. It is because we find it difficult to admit that we made a mistake. In addition, we continue to buy something because we do not have the skill to say enough is enough.

Often we see this with people who buy one brand of car, television, shoes, clothing, etc. It seems that unless the trend changes and someone else decides that there is something new to wear or eat, the probability is that you will see people buy the same brand over and over again.

It seems that social trendsetters have the power to direct our attention towards something new. We are allowing others to direct our attention, and our choices are then minimized. Take control of where your attention is directed and be sure that you know what you want to have in your life.

Focus on Establishing Emotional Balance

In essence, we believe that for some whose metabolism efficiently stores fat, it is vital to create a mental environment that is stable and secure. This is especially important for those who have a nervous disposition and are experiencing unnecessarily high states of anxiety and fear. Take the time and check how you feel when you are still. What happens? How long can your mind stay calm? What happens when you are alone? What is going on with your thinking?

Find solutions to what arises in your mind, send a clear message to your mind that you are safe and that your needs are met. Give your mind decisive instructions with genuine and sincere perspectives that your world is safe and all is well. Then your world will be just that.

Affirmations

Affirmations are dangerous, in some instances perhaps even fatal to our success. We often read about the power of affirmations and how important it is to repeat positive affirmations frequently to ourselves. Regrettably, in most cases, this can be foolhardy.

Our mind has some unusual characteristics when it comes to self-talk. It is important to understand what these are. When we tell ourselves/affirm that we are "something," we are bringing our focus of attention to that thing and prioritizing it and validating its existence.

Whilst we are affirming/confirming "something," our mind is engaged in perceiving it. Imagine someone sitting on his couch, weighing in at sixteen stone, affirming, *"I am slim"* whilst struggling to sit in comfort.

What is that person's mind likely to believe? The mind is most likely to accept what it is being told. If our mind is told we are slim, it will accept that as fact, therefore there is nothing else to be done as far as the mind is concerned.

Our mind is many things, including being minimalist. In other words, it will do the least it can to fulfill its needs. This includes duping us into believing something is happening when in fact it is just allowing us to fall into the trap of self-deception.

Affirmations need to be carefully and thoughtfully crafted. To sit in the wilderness and tell ourselves that we have fire whilst sitting in pitch darkness is lunacy. We need at least to have a spark of light to begin creating a fire. If we do not, we need to put ourselves in a place where we can create a flicker of flame, at the very least, in order to create fire.

Unless we can perceive a possibility, it does not exist. If, though, we realize that we have resources—a battery and some wire wool, and that we can connect a cable and scrape the wire wool with the other—we can start a fire.

In the same way, when we are affirming something along the lines of "I am slim and beautiful" whilst staring at a body that we dislike, what is the potential here?

The rule for affirmations is simple: there needs to be a truth, no matter how small, that fits in with your desires and expectation. For instance, we might be in a situation where we have overdone ice cream in the past. If, though, we can remember that we had said "no" to ice cream on one occasion, then we can affirm, *"I can say no to ice cream."*

In another situation, we might recall that we lost fat when we were on holiday. We may then affirm, "I lose fat." Just remember that is what happened, and then it can happen again.

Perhaps the best general affirmation that we would recommend to use is from the French psychologist Emile Cue, master of positive autosuggestions/affirmations and mantras:

"Every day in every way, I am getting better and better."

We would add that in order for the affirmation to be more potent, we need also to perceive/imagine an element of our lives where things have really got better. This is where the mind will have the added benefit and continue to fulfill the affirmation.

Perceive It, Believe It, and the Mind Will Use All Its Resources to Achieve It!

Let's consider the man sitting on his couch. What does he perceive? What is his experience at this time? What does he believe about his physical condition? It is doubtful that he believes that he is slim. Consequently, he will experience little if any change through his "I am slim" affirmation. Perhaps he will even get bigger.

Affirmations can work if they are crafted and constructed with a high degree of realism and linguistic precision. It is vital to affirm what is and not what is not.

Now, we could argue that the point is to direct the mind to what we would like to have happen in our lives. However, it is important to differentiate between affirmations and goal setting.

There is no substitute for a well-formed goal being set. Affirmations simply validate *what is* and *not what is not.* Goals direct the mind, aiming it in a particular direction with an objective in sight.

Validating what is through affirmation requires a little time to construct the right image and words. Let us assume that you are choosing to affirm that you are losing weight and changing size in the process.

Constructing an affirmation such as "I am slim and beautiful" whilst feeling fat and unable to appreciate your appearance results in perpetuating what you feel rather than what you say to yourself.

If, on the other hand, you can see that you have done something different, albeit a small thing, you could validate that through affirmation. Let's say that today you decided to skip that snack that was available to you in the office. You can then affirm that you resisted temptation, because you did. Therefore, you can affirm, "I resist temptation," and that is a truism.

When you can get into an item of clothing that you have not been able to get into for a while, you can affirm that your shape is changing. Your affirmation can be, "I am reducing my size."

So let's spell it out clearly. An affirmation needs to affirm something that is meant. If you do not mean it, then it is not true and therefore invalid. Therefore, finding something that is true and emphasizing it through affirmation is a key to weight loss. You are probably getting the idea by now.

The next step is simply an advancement of the existing affirmation. Once you have constructed an affirmation through selecting something good from the day, when you do it a second time, you can affirm, "Day by day, I eat more healthily and feel better and better." Once you have reached your desired goal, you can then confirm, "I am at the right weight and shape."

Think of affirmations simply as truisms. They are honest truths about your progress, magnified and highlighted so your mind can focus on something that you consider to be an accomplishment. Once you have set your mind to a successful outcome, like a child that needs encouragement, be kind, caring, and encouraging for more of the same. For more information on affirmations, visit our Web site.

Making Successful Changes

Often we have encountered people who have initially set out passionately on a journey that they have chosen to make. It may be a career change, a new relationship, an exercise program, something that they want out of life.

More often than not, these people end up in a place that they did not plan for. They keep repeating the same mistakes over and over again. Frustrations overcome and then they are up and at it again, only to find themselves repeating the cycle until eventually they accept the situation as unchangeable and give in to their current state.

Little if any attention is given to the planning aspect of change. Change requires the acceptance that things will be different. Change requires acceptance that we will lose something (the mind abhors loss) in the process. Equally important is to grasp that change requires planning. Most people do not set out to fail; they simply fail to plan for success. There is a lovely quote, "goals are dreams with deadlines." It really is about setting a goal and designing a successful strategy to bring it to fruition.

So what is entailed in putting together a plan? Short of reading *Change Directions*, a book about changing and designing a way forward, we would suggest taking time to specifically address your needs and wants. In other words, your objectives and your desired outcome.

Simply consider the information given to you through this book, and once you have read it and digested the information, plan your journey.

Consider the following questions and write down your answers; this will help solidify your decision-making.

Have I fully understood the situation I am in?

What is my objective?

How would I describe my objective to a person who knows nothing about weight loss (the details of a successful outcome)?

What does reaching my objective entail?

Why is it important to reach my objective?

What will happen if I do not have this objective?

What will I need to give up (lose) in gaining my objective?

What am I not prepared to give up to reach my objective?

Do you believe that you can achieve your objective? Beliefs are cornerstones of actions and outcomes. You will need to ensure that at best you are purposeful and certain that you will accomplish your objective.

Based on past attempts, what will be different this time?

On a scale of 1 (being low) and 10 (being high) how do you rate your chances of success? If you score yourself less than 10, what would need to happen for you to be a 10?

Based on the knowledge contained within this book, your target size, your resources, when do you need to reach your target weight/size? You need a realistic timeline that is achievable. You need to pick that date yourself.

Setting an objective is critical to any outcome. Not having an objective often results in unspecified outcomes that may deplete further your will, your resources, and your self-image. Look at past outcomes and explore what did not happen and how it was possible for it not to happen.

When will I be ready to start to deal with weight control, start with a plan, and stick to the plan until successful completion?

In order to design a way forward, there needs to be something in it for us. If what's in it for us is meager in comparison to the instant gratification of poor quality food choices, it is unrealistic to believe that that we are going to engage with the process of changing our weight.

The value for losing weight needs to be greater than the sacrifice involved in getting there.

Unless we can see/hear that the benefits are substantial, it is unlikely that we will get past the first few days of getting into the program. A halfhearted attempt will be made, and then challenges will most likely beat us.

Just Do It

There are those who best function when they do not think about it, they "just do it"—no thinking about anything else, just get into a new routine and do it. No time to think about it, no doubt, no discussions, no getting on the scales every minute, no anything. Really simple, just understand the desired weight or size that we need to get to and do it. Just be focused on doing what you need to do.

By hook or by crook, just get on with it. No whining, no moaning, no attention seeking, no praise, no applause, until your target weight/size is reached and maintained. This, for some people, is the best solution to getting there.

Stand Tall

Walk your talk. Communicate to others if you can about how well you feel about your newfound interest in your physical and mental state. Avoid judgment and criticism. Whenever you make a judgment of another person, you are revealing your fears and heading towards attracting those fears.

If you cannot say anything nice about yourself, then say nothing. If you can say something nice without it sounding arrogant, then praise your accomplishments. Remember, what you are focused on is what you are asking for.

Avoid "Don't"

The law of reversed effort disables the mind from seeking anything other than the thing that it is focused upon. How this works is simple: the more we say "don't," the more the mind does.

As an example of this, we will give you an instruction to do something: please don't think about a little pink piggy with a red ribbon bouncing on a cloud.

The probability is that you will have imagined the little piggy. The more you tell yourself "don't," the more you likely do. Don't think about the answer to 2 + 2; not easy to ignore the number 4. What this means in terms of weight loss is that we are very easily able to trap ourselves in a situation that results in our being unable to escape from our own thinking.

The following examples might give clarity and solutions to these phenomena. "I don't want to put more weight on" creates an image of weight being put on. You may have discovered that telling someone, "Don't put any ketchup on it," all too often results in getting it with ketchup.

The sentence needs to be constructed in such a way that gives the instruction of what to do, not what not to do. In the previous example, we could say, "I would like it plain, thank you." That is a direct and clear instruction.

Additionally, when it comes to self-talk, we do need to be extremely cautious of words and phrases such as "I ought to," "I should," "I must," etc.—words that imply that you are forced to do something that you do not want to do.

There are consequences when our language mismatches our needs. In this instance, we are seeking to be empowered and exhibit confidence in our abilities to start and maintain a healthy diet. On one hand, we are saying we want to do this, and on the other, we say "we ought" to do this. There is an implied suggestion here. "We ought to be able to do this" is suggesting that that we are not going to; rather, we are going to do something else. In the same way, when we say "I should," we are implying "but I am not going to." Take caution when using words that disempower.

Keep your words strong, positive, and empowering to your needs and wants. Once you have made your decision to start, just get on with it. No ifs or buts, just do it. If it is your decision to find excuses to not do it, then at the very least say so and accept that this is how life works for you. Be happy with your decisions, as this will add volumes of confidence about them.

There are several such oddities about our mental operating system, and it is prudent to consider words like *try, wish, hope,* etc. There is a small book listed in the resource section to help.

Those Around You

The loving and well-intentioned person is often the last one we would perceive as a threat to our success. We can so easily be scuppered by well-meaning and in some cases loving, caring individuals who think they can alleviate the early days of discomfort that we need to surpass while we adapt to healthy eating.

Those who inadvertently scupper our success by saying "I bought you this little tub of ice cream because you are doing so well and I thought you deserve a little treat" well, we could thank them for that, then sit and destroy a day's vigilance in about ten minutes.

We might see their face nervously giving the tub to us and feeling that if we are to reject their offer, they will feel hurt or get offended and we might lose them as a friend. Often they themselves are imagining what we are going through and cannot help but to see if they can alleviate the pain they perceive we are experiencing.

Nice thought, though it's not what's good for us. What is important is to accept that these mostly well-meaning people have a need to do good, for they perceive you as suffering.

In the event that such a delivery is made, it would help to cap the flow of this unwanted generosity. An error is to accept their kindness and to make out that you are enjoying the treat. Pause here, consider the message you are sending your mind. This could be suggesting that other people's feelings are more important than your health.

Care for Yourself

It is imperative that you believe you are important enough to care about. Self-worth and self-esteem play a vital part in the final outcome of your weight loss and your life generally.

It is unlikely that you would have purchased this book if you did not care to some degree about yourself. Often we tend to feel embarrassed to acknowledge that we care about ourselves sincerely. Here we are not talking about those whose insecurities are masked by illusions of grandeur, but a genuine care for oneself.

Sympathize with your body's strengths and not weaknesses. There is a tendency for some to focus on their weaknesses. You may have met some who seem to go on about how difficult it is for them—a constant whine, a struggle, a chore, fixated on the challenge as if it is a problem and something they are being forced to do.

The Decision to Change

The bottom line is that it is *all about choice*. No, we do not have to do anything about our weight. We can stay big, and that's that. At no time is anyone holding a gun to our head. The talent is the choices we make. We can choose to see doing this as an unpleasant task, or as an opportunity, or we can be indifferent.

Common sense would tell us that seeing it as a problem will make it a problem, and seeing it as an opportunity will more likely bring opportunities and make it more interesting and even fun.

Some people struggle with disappointment and consequently prepare themselves with an attitude of impending doom. The chemical effects of stress on the body can further damage the degree of reparation to our system. For those who have a propensity to negative thoughts, we would recommend the *"just do it"* attitude.

Making decisions is hard work for the mind. It takes a lot of energy. It is tiring. In fact, at times it can be so exhausting that we give the right to choose away, so that we do not have to make decisions.

As mentioned in this book, the whole process is easily simplified by the mind's ability to create patterns of behavior that become routines and act as instructions that require little or no attention from us. This is a good thing so long as the pattern has a healthy, life-giving outcome.

Regrettably, this is often not the case. In fact, there are times that we simply give up and thereby give in to old patterns that we continue to follow irrespective of their result.

It comes down to the fact that to make good quality decisions requires information, analysis, and benefit evaluation. Those of you who use a process such as the Six Hats, created by Dr. Edward de Bono, may realize how valuable the ability to make quick, quality decisions is by reducing thinking time to a minimum.

Decisions about how you want to feel as you journey through life necessitate that you think about the lifestyle required to facilitate this. That requires a conscious awareness of what is and what needs to be in order to "as best you can" get into a lifestyle that works for you.

Challenge your assumptions and fight off the natural tendency to accept the status quo, and you will stand a chance of minimizing the damage done to your experience of life.

Let us be very clear about one thing: if the mind has been programmed or duped into behaving in particular ways, *it is our responsibility to break the program.* It may often be the case that we need help, perhaps in the form of therapy, counseling, nutritional assistance, or simply a witness. A witness is someone who will act as a mentor and help ensure we stay the course.

None of this will matter unless we decide and act. It is as simple as that. Decide, plan, and act. If at first you don't succeed, find another way. It really is all about correct persistence.

Avoid Playing the Victim

Something that can thwart our progress is when we fall into the "poor me" or "it's not fair" game. This game is designed to ensure that we stay stuck through relinquishing our personal power, on the basis that something is out of our control and that we can do nothing about it.

If you find yourself in this place, pause and take some time to reflect on your attitude and how it affects your thinking and behavior. Check to see if you are using this type of mind-set to defend an attitude that allows you to eat unhealthy or inferior foods.

The question that perhaps may help is: "Which means what, exactly?" If it's unfair, so what? If it makes you feel a victim, then realize that you are unlikely to change anything. If you are angry about it, then do something about it. In reality, as far as nature is concerned, there is no such thing as "unfair"; it is just what it is. No more, no less.

Deletion, Generalization, and Distortion

The ways in which our minds operate have been better understood since the development of neurolinguistics in the 1970s (Bandler and Grindler). How the mind processes information is crucial to understand when it comes to maintaining stable patterns.

There are three processes that the mind uses to keep things known and certain. These are deletion, generalization and distortion. These are necessary in order to maintain stability in the way we see the world.

Deletion

The mind deletes information by being selective about what it allows us to see/hear and remember. This is perhaps the most subtle of the three, as it is not easy to know what has been deleted. You might recall a conversation with someone where he or she insists that something was not said. Deletions occur across all areas of life. In other words, it is not exclusive to just words; we also delete other types of information.

You may recall someone saying that she has only had a small lunch that day, yet you might be aware of the fact that during the day you were there when she had eaten a nut with honey bar and a slice of pie in the afternoon.

Conveniently deleting what does not fit in with what we would like to believe is common. One of the ways to combat this is to keep a food diary. There is less chance of deletion occurring, and we we are more likely to double our weight control success.

In the same way we can delete what we have consumed, we delete other information. This can include deleting positive actions and disregarding our accomplishments.

This erodes and dilutes our personal power and may consequently leave us unable to sustain our efforts.

There is little chance of realizing deletions after the fact. Once the deletion has occurred, we no longer have instant access as with other memories. The cure is awareness and alertness.

Some may not have noticed that three paragraphs above this one, the word "we" was repeated twice consecutively. This is deletion in action.

Generalization

Another wonderful ability is that the mind will generalize information so that it can normalize situations without the need to change beliefs.

We might hear someone say "you're looking great." If we do not believe that about ourselves, we are likely to think, "She says that to everyone," and thereby generalize and depersonalize the statement.

Generalizations can be used constructively and destructively. An example of how marketers use generalization might be, "Our research* shows that our KAKA berries produce better results than any other berries." (*Research stats: 168 people were asked to participate in our test, and eighty-six people reported a benefit with KAKA berries.)

Those who bother to look closely at the research will see that only slightly more than half the subjects of the research noted a benefit, yet the advertisers generalize the results to make a more impressive impact.

Here is another type of generalization. How often are we likely to hear someone say: "Well, I don't believe that it is bad for you; the fact is that I know people who have eaten like this all their lives and nothing happened to them."

We can generalize about our progress through looking at the big picture and reporting that we are accomplishing more using our new method of weight loss. Have you sat down to a meal as prescribed and realized that by preparing and consuming quality food and being aware of the pleasure of this meal, we can generalize that "the new approach I am using to lose fat weight is a pleasure"? This is an example of positive generalization.

Distortion

As a way of maintaining our beliefs, our mind utilizes its ability to make things fit in with what it knows and understands. The implication of this is vast. We are able to see a situation and bend it to fit with what we want to see or hear.

We may report that we had a little treat on the way home when in fact we had a bowl of ice cream. We distort information to enhance our experience in order that it is in keeping with our beliefs.

In some instances, we do not see the evidence in front of us. Our ability to distort may make the journey to reducing our weight longer and even prevent it.

The cure is to be factual about what is said and what is experienced. There is no space for naivety in our quest for control of our body. This book will help to identify and correct many of the misconceptions about how the body processes food.

Planning Ahead

Planning ahead is important, especially when you begin to change your nutritional habits. Having the right foods in stock and on hand can be the difference between keeping to your healthy eating plan and stopping by the convenience store and grabbing a readymade sandwich, a bar of chocolate, or bag of chips.

So keep your fridge well stocked, full of healthy and tasty foods, and keep in mind what day you will next need to go shopping to restock. When you are running low on healthy and fresh foods make your next food shop a scheduling priority.

Keep an emergency backup supply of tinned tuna or salmon and some frozen or tinned vegetables on hand in case any scheduling issues mean you have to delay your shop by an evening or a day. This ensures that you can keep on track, rather than using a lack of healthy food on hand as an excuse to grab some junk.

Also, plan ahead in thinking what you'll be eating for breakfast, lunch, dinner, and any snacks you may want to keep on hand tomorrow. Having a plan means you will get to where you want to go rather than being sidetracked or going off path.

Keeping a Food Diary

As well as planning ahead, another useful technique to use when you are first changing your nutritional habits is keeping a food diary.

Over a typical week, keep a food diary. Note down everything you eat and when. This will make you more aware of the good and bad nutritional choices you make. It will highlight areas that need to be changed. Some people may have an initial resistance to keeping a food diary, stating reasons like, "Oh, I don't have time to do that," or "I don't need to write it down, I can remember what I eat."

The first reason given is weak; we can tell you that at the absolute maximum, it will take you thirty seconds to note down what you've just eaten for a main meal, and for a snack it will take all of ten seconds. In less than two minutes a day, you will be able to keep an accurate track of what you are eating.

Remember we are not asking you to note down grams of food consumed or to look up and add up calories—there is absolutely no need to do that whatsoever, ever again. Just note down what you ate; e.g., breakfast: 3 eggs scrambled, 2 tomatoes, handful of blueberries; snack: slice of cheese. That is as much detail as you require.

Make sure you note down everything that passes your lips during the entire day. Leave nothing out, especially if you do slip up. Many people, especially the ones who say, "I don't need to write it down, I can remember," have a tendency of forgetting the unhealthy things they ate. When you ask them, they'll say "Oh, yeah, really good day today, healthy breakfast, lunch, and dinner."

What their minds will have conveniently omitted is the chocolate bar they had between breakfast and lunch or the serving of pasta they had alongside their otherwise healthy dinner. They are not omitting it to be deceitful, but the human mind is very good at distortion, deletion, and generalization.

So keep your food diary on you, in your handbag, or in a pocket, and just take a moment to note down what you eat straight after you've eaten it. This isn't something you'll have to do forever either. Perhaps for the first month of your new way of eating and then occasionally for a week every now and then if you hit a sticking point in your weight loss. It'll really draw your focus and attention back to what you are actually eating and exactly where you need to make changes.

We've seen it time and time again with clients; those who keep a food diary outperform those who don't every time in terms of weight loss. It can mean the difference between losing two pounds or a kilogram a week and breaking even or increasing weight. If a client ever goes off track, all we have to do is produce a food diary and their weight is soon dropping off again.

Scientific research has backed up the value of keeping a food diary. A study published in the *American Journal of Preventive Medicine* discovered that people who keep a food diary whilst dieting lose on average twice as much weight as those who do not. Now surely results like that are worth a two-minute time investment per day.[1]

ೞ

IN CONCLUSION:

- Planning ahead for your food shopping and what you will eat tomorrow is empowering yourself and brings greater stability and reduces fear in your mind. Inform your mind through your actions and planning that there will always be quality food available for you.

- Keep your language constructive rather than destructive. Keep it simple by adjusting your responses to "I can, I need, I want" and "Thank you…no," as well as "That's not possible" when you have no need. These responses, once mastered, will further direct your mind to your intentions.

- Be vigilant of your mind's distortions by seeking to get all the facts. Be cautious of what your mind deletes, especially concerning your food intake. A food diary can help to minimize the possibility of mentally deleting what you have consumed. Generalizations can excuse and cover up all sorts of misdemeanors, so be aware. Telling yourself, "Well, my friend is on a diet, and she is eating kaka berries," so as to make it okay for you to eat them, is not clever.

- Focus on extracting all the nutritional information from this book and begin focusing on making positive changes to your dietary habits. Become aware of the foods you are buying and eating.

- You always have choice. Exercise your right to choose to eat well; after all, your body may not be the one that you would have designed for yourself, but it is not a trash can.

PART TWO

"*Success will never be a big step in the future, success is a small step taken just now.*"

Jonatan Martensson

Chapter 9.
The ONE Diet "In a Nutshell"

HOW TO EAT HEALTHILY AND LOSE WEIGHT

*The key to eating well and maximizing your weight loss is to combine a protein/fat option (1), with vegetables or salad (2), cooked in and/or dressed with a healthy fat (3), from the **DO EAT** list on the next page, at every main meal.*

For convenience you may choose to omit vegetables/salad at breakfast.

It is best to eliminate or at least minimize between-meal snacks. It will serve you best if any snacks you do have consist of an item from the five categories of healthy snacks (4) or a combination, e.g., sliced apple with cheddar cheese, or blueberries with whole cream. Selecting items from the healthy snack options is also a great way to create a quick and easy breakfast.

*Unless noted otherwise, you do not need to limit your consumption of the foods listed in categories 1- 4 of the **DO EAT** list.*

DO EAT

1. Protein/Fat—Choose from this list: beef, lamb, fish, game, goat, pork, poultry and eggs (if you can, source pastured pork, poultry and eggs as they have a healthier fat profile than the factory reared or grain fed types). Eat between 8–16 ounces (250–500 grams) of animal foods per day.

2. Vegetables/Salad—Almost all vegetables and salad are acceptable. *The only exceptions are:* potatoes, sweet potatoes, yams, parsnips, cassava, and sweet corn. These vegetables are may be too starchy for many people during the process of losing weight. You can however, include these vegetables in a dish from time to time.

3. Healthy Fats—Use these fats for cooking; butter (ideally pastured butter from cows fed grass), lard, ghee and unrefined virgin coconut oil. Use extra virgin olive oil as a salad dressing if you enjoy the flavor.

4. Healthy Snacks:

a) High quality cured meats, continental sausages, and cold sliced meats that have no added sugars, carbohydrates, or excess chemical preservatives. To be acceptable, a sausage ideally needs to have 90 percent or higher meat content with less than two grams of carbohydrates per sausage or serving. The nutritional information label will show this information.

b) Approved fruits—Limit to one to two portions per day whilst focusing on weight loss. *These fruits are particularly good for us during weight loss:* all varieties of fresh berries, cherries, apples, pears, apricots, peaches, plums, kiwi, pomegranates, figs, prunes, bananas, and grapefruit.

Minimize or, ideally, cut out altogether these fruits whilst reducing your weight, as they have higher sugar content: grapes, watermelons, melons, dates, mangoes, papayas, pineapples, nectarines, oranges, tangerines, and all dried fruits.

c) Whole (full-fat) cream and/or coconut milk—Ensure it is a pure cream or coconut milk with no added sweeteners/sugars.

d) Approved nuts—Choose from this list: almonds, walnuts, macadamias, pistachios, hazelnuts, pecans, pine nuts, brazils. If you enjoy the taste of any of these nuts, have an occasional palmful or add them to a salad.

e) Approved cheeses—Mature and hard cheeses (as they contain less lactose (milk sugar) and their protein content is more digestible than soft cheeses) including: cheddar, gorgonzola, parmesan, gouda, edam, emmental and gruyere. Soft cheeses are acceptable if you find they cause you no digestive distress. Avoid processed cheeses altogether.

WHAT TO AVOID

In addition to eating healthy foods from the previous list, it is important for your health and weight loss to avoid the following:

1. Grains—Cereal grains, whole grains, refined grains, flours, or products that contain grains—pasta, bread, breakfast cereals, pastries, biscuits, crackers, pies and other bakery goods.

Rice is a partial exception to this rule as it is a nongluten grain and has far fewer inflammatory antinutrients than the gluten grains like wheat. The antinutrient phytin, which is present in the bran of brown rice and wild rice is milled and polished away from the grain during the process used to produce white rice. All remaining antinutrients in white rice are denatured and made safe by exposure to heat (e.g. during cooking). A small portion of white rice may be included as a side to a main meal occasionally during the weight loss process. Unsweetened puffed rice paired with a *small* amount of half-and-half, half cream or whole (full-fat) milk may make a suitable breakfast for some people.

White rice may slow or halt weight loss for some individuals, if this is the case you may need to eliminate rice altogether for a time.

2. Sugars And Sweeteners—Foods and drinks that contain added sugars and sweeteners, including table sugar, sucrose, dextrose, fructose, high fructose corn syrup, rice syrup, glucose, artificial sweeteners (saccharine, sucralose, aspartame, etc.), and so on. (These sweeteners are also often present in ready meals, cakes, biscuits, jams, confectionary, desserts, sodas, soft drinks, sports/energy drinks, etc.).

3. Unhealthy Fats—Vegetable/grain/seed and nut; oils, fats, and spreads. Hydrogenated oil/fat, partially hydrogenated oil/fat, trans fats, and interesterified fats. Also, avoid products containing these fats; check the nutritional label.

4. Altered Fat Level Products—All "low-fat," "fat-free," and "reduced-fat" products. This includes semi-skimmed and skimmed milk, low-fat yoghurts, low-fat cheeses, etc.

5. Legumes And Pulses—Soybeans, soya, and all soy products, all mature beans and peas (including dried beans and peas), lentils and peanuts.

Edible immature beans and peas, many of which can be eaten in their pods, are however healthy and perfectly acceptable, including: green beans, french beans, runner beans, string beans, green peas, snap peas, sugarsnap peas, mangetout and snow peas. Treat these immature beans and peas as you would vegetables.

6. Fruit Juices—All fruit juices, as they contain far too much sugar.

7. Junk Food In General—Ready meals, microwave meals, crisps, chocolate, crackers, fast food/junk food, soft drinks, etc.

8. Processed Meat—Sausages and other processed meats that have been filled out with carbohydrates and sugars.

9. High-Carbohydrate Alcoholic Drinks—Beer and lager, cider, sweet wines and fortified wines (port, sherry, dessert wines).

By cutting out the items in this list, you will have eliminated the foods and ingredients that are responsible for triggering weight gain. Moreover, you will have taken some of the most beneficial steps possible to improving your long-term health.

Chapter 10.
The ONE Diet in Six Steps

A STEP-BY-STEP GUIDE

Follow the six steps in this chapter to maximize your understanding of The ONE Diet and ensure your success. In addition, your progress will largely be determined by your ability to cut out the foods mentioned in the AVOID lists throughout this chapter.

STEP ONE: BREAKFAST

A lot is often made in nutrition circles about how important having breakfast is, to the degree that its importance has become exaggerated. The likelihood is that when you have breakfast, you will have been in a fasted state for at least eight hours, probably longer.

Metabolically, most people could quite easily last until lunch to break their overnight fast and doing so can benefit weight loss.

What is important if you are going to eat breakfast is what you consume. Most people, unfortunately, reach straight for that box of unhealthy grain-loaded breakfast cereal, which is about the worst thing someone hoping to lose weight could possibly do.

Inputting your system with an excessive amount of refined carbohydrate is going to stimulate increased hunger over the following hours—potentially causing a midmorning dip in energy and sugar cravings.

If you do eat breakfast select an option from the list below or mix and match items from the list to create your own delicious breakfasts.

The Healthy Breakfast Choices

Eggs scrambled in butter (add some smoked salmon or bacon for variety)

Boiled eggs

Omelet

Bacon fried in butter. Any meat is fine actually. If you have the taste and the time for cooking a steak or piece of chicken for breakfast, you may do so.

Approved sausage or continental sausage—check that it is very low in carbohydrates and *not* low on meat or packed with filler carbohydrate. To be acceptable, a sausage needs to be 90 percent or higher in meat content with less than two grams of carbohydrates per sausage/serving.

Cold sliced meats

Approved fruits—in particular, all fresh berries; other good choices include cherries, apples, pears, apricots, peaches, plums, kiwi, pomegranates, figs, prunes, bananas, and grapefruit. *Remember to limit fruit to one or two portions a day whilst reducing your weight.*

Natural full fat yoghurt (e.g., Greek yoghurt)

Full fat coconut milk (check that no sweeteners have been added)

Full fat cream

Approved cheeses— mature and hard cheeses, including: cheddar, gorgonzola, parmesan, gouda, edam, emmental and gruyere. Soft cheeses are acceptable if you find they cause you no digestive distress. Avoid processed cheeses altogether.

Approved nuts—good choices are almonds, walnuts, macadamias, pistachios, hazelnuts, pecans, pine nuts, brazils.

Unsweetened puffed rice with a *small* amount of half-and-half, half cream or whole (full-fat) milk. *This option may need to be an occasional choice or even curtailed altogether for some people during weight loss due to the quantity of starch and presence of lactose (milk sugar).*

Avoid

Cereals and mueslis

Porridge

Toast/bread

Breakfast bars/cereal bars, etc.

Croissants and other pastries

Jams, conserves, and marmalades

Fruit juice

Typical store-bought sausages (containing too much cheap filler carbohydrate)

Skimmed and semi-skimmed milk (a very small amount of full fat milk may be fine if you can tolerate lactose)

Soya milk

Grain milks

Added sugar or other sweeteners

Pulses, legumes and baked beans

STEP TWO: THE MAIN MEALS

Lunch and dinner are essentially the cornerstones of our diet and a great chance for us to fill up on healthy, energy-sustaining foods that will reinforce our weight loss progress. Unfortunately, in the modern world they are usually yet another opportunity for people to serve their addiction to sugars and refined carbohydrates.

Remember to combine a protein/fat source with some healthy vegetable carbohydrates and to prepare and/or dress your meal with a healthy fat (healthy fats for cooking and dressing are listed in Step Three).

Healthy Main Meal Choices

Protein/Fat Choices:

Beef, lamb, game, goat, pork and poultry

Eggs

Fish

Prawns/shrimp

Offal

Approved cheeses

Avocado

Approved nuts—to add to salads, etc.

Healthy Carbohydrate Choices:

All vegetables *(except those mentioned in the AVOID list)*

Salad greens and leaves, watercress, rocket, spinach, baby spinach, kale, etc.

Eggplant/aubergines

Zucchini/courgettes

Peppers

Onions

Mushrooms

Tomatoes

Asparagus

Hot peppers

Edible immature beans and peas: green beans, french beans, runner beans, string beans, green peas, snap peas, sugarsnap peas, mangetout and snow peas

Sea vegetables, seaweed, etc.

Approved fruit—*remember to limit fruit to one or two portions a day while your goal is to reduce your weight*

Avoid

All cereal grains and products made from cereal grains (whole grain products included)

All flour and products containing flour (except coconut flour)

Sweet corn and all corn-based products

Pasta

Noodles (noodles made purely from rice, with no other grains listed in the ingredients can be treated as rice: see below)

Rice (a small portion of white rice, the healthiest of the grains, *may* be added to a dish *occasionally* during the weight loss process)

Bread, buns, rolls, sandwiches, crackers, tortillas, etc.

Pastries and pies

Pizza

Ready meals (especially those with added sugar/dextrose/glucose/high fructose corn syrup, etc.)

French fries/chips

Fast food, junk food—the usual suspects

Battered foods

Sugars, sweeteners, and sugar substitutes

"Low-fat"/"fat-free"/"reduced- fat" products

Soy and soy-based products

Pulses, legumes, dried peas and beans, peanuts and lentils

Baked beans

Typical filler- based sausages

Sweets/desserts (they are usually high in sugar/sweeteners)

Skimmed, semi-skimmed and "low-fat" milk

In Addition, Avoid Or At Least Exercise Caution With These Vegetables

For effective fat loss, the vegetables listed below often need to be minimized and for some people cut out all together. For those who have attained their ideal weight, the starchy vegetables listed below *may* be reintroduced into the diet.

All varieties of white potatoes

Sweet potatoes

Yams

Parsnips

Cassava

STEP THREE: FATS AND OILS

Healthy Fats And Oils

Fats And Oils For Cooking

Butter, ideally pastured butter (from cows fed grass)

Ghee

Lard

Unrefined coconut oil

Oil For Dressing And Drizzling

Extra virgin olive oil

Avoid These Fats And Oils

Margarine and all other "fake butter"/"fake oil" spreads (including those derived from soy, olive, sunflower, and other vegetable oils). This includes spreads that are a combination of real butter with a vegetable oil.

Any fat or oil that is hydrogenated, partially hydrogenated, or that contains trans- fats or interesterified fats.

Vegetable, seed, grain and nut oils, including sunflower oil, soy oil, etc. Note that there are now olive oils on the market that have been blended with another vegetable oil; these are also to be avoided.

More On Fats And Oils

Make sure all your fats and oils are unrefined whenever possible.

Good quality butter can be used for medium-high-heat cooking and frying.

For high-heat cooking up to temperatures of around 375°F/190°C, the best choices are ghee, lard, clarified butter, and unrefined coconut oil, which are amongst the most heat resilient of fats.

Another oil you may choose to cook with is unrefined virgin red palm oil (steer clear of the refined versions, which do not have the same health benefits). It is good for high-temperature baking and cooking, as it is stable and very heat resistant, having a high smoke point of 437°F /225°C.

Red palm oil does have a strong taste, and if you are going to use it for cooking, we would suggest trialing it to see if you enjoy its taste and what foods it complements for you.

If you can, source West African red palm oil, as this is the most eco-friendly location for production of this healthy oil.

Cooking Advice

Rather than heating up your cooking pan, then adding your cooking fat, put the fat in an unheated pan and gradually heat the fat up to help avoid oxidization of the healthy fats.

STEP FOUR: SNACKS AND DESSERTS

This is the one area where most people who are overweight or putting on excess weight really come unstuck. So many of the convenience snacks and foods that are available to us undo any chance of weight loss. It is usually best to get out of the habit of snacking altogether. This is a key area in which you will need to focus on making changes.

If you find initially you just cannot go between main meals without an occasional snack the list that follows consists of healthy, nutritious foods that will help you to stay on track and losing weight.

Healthy Between-Meal Snacks

Hard-boiled eggs

Canned tuna, salmon, and sardines

Approved cheeses

Full-fat double cream

Coconut milk (ensure this has no added sweeteners)

Natural full-fat yoghurt (e.g., Greek yoghurt)

Smoked salmon

A tablespoon of coconut oil

Cold, sliced meat

Cold prawns

Avocado

Tomatoes

Olives

Approved fruit—*remember, whilst aiming to lose weight, restrict fruit intake to one or two portions a day*

Sliced vegetables

Pickles

Beef jerky

Dark chocolate (85 percent cocoa or higher)

Approved nuts

Pure puffed rice cakes or pure rice crackers with a healthy fat spread on top

Delicious Desserts

Fruit with full-fat cream

Natural full-fat yoghurt, to which you can add your own chopped fresh fruit

Avoid

Regular chocolate bars/chocolate

Cereal bars, cereal and nut bars, fruit 'n' nut bars, etc.

Sweets/candy/confectionary

Protein powders

Diet shakes and diet bars

Crisps

Chips

French fries

Bakery/patisserie goods—cakes, pastries, sausage rolls, bread, buns, rolls, pies, donuts, pizza slices, etc.

Biscuits

Breakfast cereals

Crackers

Peanuts, cashews, sweet chestnuts, and any nuts that have been roasted (commercial roasting temperatures turn the oils and fats bad)

Candied or sugar-coated nuts

Sweetened popcorn

Ice cream

Sports/energy bars

Junk/fast food

Pretzels

Bagels

Noodles

Any manufactured food labeled "fat-free" or "low-fat"

Chocolate Lover?

What many people mean when they say "I like chocolate" is actually "I like sugar and milk solids with a hint of chocolate flavor." Natural chocolate is an acceptable treat. When we are talking chocolate, we mean real dark chocolate, which is around 85 percent cocoa solids.

Dark chocolate makes for a reasonable treat in moderation for those who enjoy the taste of real chocolate. If you are used to eating milk chocolate, we grant you, this is going to take some getting used to. However, over a period of several weeks, as your taste buds adapt to less sugar in your diet, some of you will begin to enjoy the rich taste of quality dark chocolate as an occasional treat.

STEP FIVE: INGREDIENTS, SAUCES, CONDIMENTS, HERBS AND SPICES

These Ingredients Are Healthy

Full-fat unsweetened coconut milk

Coconut flour

Herbs, fresh if possible (dried if not): coriander, parsley, dill, chives, basil, thyme, rosemary, coriander, etc.

Unrefined organic sea salt

Peppercorns (to grind)

Spices: chili, cumin, paprika, turmeric, cinnamon, garam masala, curry powder, etc.

Ginger

Tomato puree

Vinegars, e.g., balsamic vinegar, white wine vinegar, raw unfiltered cider vinegar

Full-fat homemade mayonnaise (without the vegetable oils used in commercial mayonnaise)

Sour cream

Crème fraiche

Chili sauce

Oyster sauce

Mustards

Dark chocolate (85 percent cocoa or higher)

Avoid

All flours (except coconut flour)

Refined white table salt

Sauces that have added sugar (most commercial ones do—e.g., ketchup, barbeque sauce, etc.)

Added sugar or other sweeteners

STEP SIX: DRINKS

Drinks To Enjoy

Water

Water with a squeeze of fresh orange, lemon, or lime

Coffee

Tea, hot or iced

Herbal teas or iced herbal teas

Cocoa (Dutch-processed cocoa in the United States) made with pure unsweetened cocoa powder (which will ideally have only two listed ingredients: cocoa powder and an acidity regulator like potassium carbonate). Add cream or coconut milk and water to achieve your preferred consistency and taste.

Avoid

Soft drinks, sweet drinks, colas, sodas, and carbonated drinks (including low-sugar, artificially sweetened versions)

Artificially flavored and/or sweetened mineral waters

"Sports" or "energy" drinks

Skimmed/ semi-skimmed or "low-fat" milk

Sugary coffee-based drinks, like those sold at high street coffee house chains

Protein shakes and meal replacement drinks

Fruit juice (fruit juices are nearly as sugary as soft drinks)

Sweet milk-based drinks, milk shakes

Hot chocolate (often has added sugars)

Beer and lager

Cider

Sweet wines and fortified wines (port, sherry, dessert wines, etc.)

Premixed sweet alcoholic drinks

Drinks with added sugar or other sweeteners

Is Dairy Healthy For Me?

Dairy products seem to be fine for some people and not so beneficial for others, and it largely comes down to the natural sugar contained in milk, called lactose, and additionally the dairy protein, casein. Those who are lactose intolerant obviously need to avoid milk.

Ghee, butter, and full-fat cheese contain no lactose, and full-fat cream contains only a very small amount. All of these options are likely to be fine even for those who are lactose intolerant.

Half-and-half or half cream, Jersey/Guernsey "Gold Top" milk, and regular whole (full-fat) milk contain lactose in sufficient quantities that they need to be avoided by those who are lactose intolerant. The rest of us can experiment to see how these products affect us, and if we enjoy consuming them. We recommend that they are used minimally—e.g., in recipes, or added occasionally to hot drinks rather than as a consumed as a drink by themselves, particularly whilst on a weight reduction diet.

Milk and cream that have not been pasteurized or only minimally pasteurized are better for us than brands that are labeled as homogenized, filtered, ultrafiltered, microfiltered, and ultrapasteurized or ultra-heat treated.

The closer the product is to nature, the better it is for us.

Milk, has been marketed to the public as being a good source of calcium. Calcium however, is often better absorbed from other sources, such as broccoli, leafy greens, salmon, and sardines.

Goat dairy can be a suitable alternative to cow's milk, if you enjoy the taste, as it contains less lactose and less casein—in fact, it is more similar to the nutritional profile of human breast milk.

The reasons to avoid low-fat milk and low-fat dairy products:

There is a greater percentage of sugar in terms of the sugar to protein/fat ratio in reduced-fat dairy products, which is not good or healthy for us in terms of weight loss.

Additionally, when the fat content in dairy products has been reduced, the number of fat-soluble vitamins, particularly vitamins A and D, is also reduced. Without the fat-soluble vitamins found naturally in milk and dairy, our bodies struggle to effectively utilize the protein and minerals contained in dairy products.

Caffeine Counting?

Some older nutritional advice suggests that drinking coffee and tea does not count as water intake as they are diuretics, meaning they can make you excrete water. Coffee and tea are, however, very mild diuretics, and the notion that you will have a net loss of water by drinking them is simply incorrect, unless you consume copious amounts of them. So fret not, because drinking tea and coffee does count as water intake and will hydrate you.

Caffeinated beverages are fine in moderation in a healthy diet. Moderation means up to around 300 grams of caffeine per day. To give you a basis on which to plan your caffeine consumption, here are some typical amounts of caffeine in our approved caffeinated drinks:

Coffee (average cup)—100 mg

Black tea (average cup)—50 mg

Green tea (average cup)—30 mg

White tea (average cup)—20 mg

Herbal tea—0 mg

If you have been used to adding sugar or sweeteners to your tea and coffee, you will need to stop doing so. If you absolutely must sweeten your beverages, use raw honey or traditional natural maple syrup (avoid varieties with added sugars or sweeteners, though—check the label!). Be careful to minimize and not go overboard, as they still have a high sugar load. If you can do without, leave them out! We would suggest you work towards cutting even these natural sweeteners out over time anyway *and some people may need to do so to ensure successful weight loss.*

Unrefined coconut oil can work well as a flavor enhancer in coffee (instead of a sweetener) if you enjoy the taste of coconut; it is also a good way to have more of this healthy oil in your diet.

The Importance Of Hydration

The human body requires water to function, and water does so much for us; it helps keep the body's temperature in equilibrium, it helps our digestive system, and it provides an important function on the cellular level as a lubricator and shock absorber.

Keep yourself well hydrated by drinking approved liquids throughout the day.

Alcohol

Here's some good news for those of you who enjoy consuming alcohol in moderation. Alcohol needn't be completely off the menu even when your goal is to lose weight. So long as we avoid the excessively high carbohydrate and sugary "junk" alcoholic drinks, a serving or two a day of the right kind of alcoholic beverages is fine.

Remember that overindulgence and binges, even on the relatively low carbohydrate choices below, could set you back on your weight loss goals. If binges are a regular thing, losing weight will become far more challenging than it need be. As with most good things, moderation really does rule when it comes to alcohol.

Here's a list of our top choices:

Approved Alcoholic Drinks—Yes, There Are Such Things!

From a health and weight loss perspective, we suggest that you limit yourself to one or two servings of alcoholic drinks per day. With that said, here is our list of approved alcoholic drinks:

Red wine—very low in carbohydrates—around 1 gram per serving

Dry white wine—still low in carbohydrates—around 2 grams per serving

Whisky/scotch—virtually zero carbohydrates

Brandy/cognac—virtually zero carbohydrates

White rum—virtually zero carbohydrates

Gin—virtually zero carbohydrates

Tequila—virtually zero carbohydrates

Vodka—virtually zero carbohydrates

True low carbohydrate beer/ultralight beer—essentially what you are looking for is a beer that comes in with around 2.5–3.5 grams of carbohydrates per 12 ounces or 350 ml. Be careful, though; not all beers advertised as "light" are low in carbohydrates. By the way, regular beer comes in at 9–15 grams of carbohydrates per serving, and many so-called "light" beers come in at 7–12 grams (that's four times more carbohydrates than the true low carbohydrate beers).

To be truly low carbohydrate, a beer definitely needs to have fewer than 7 grams of carbohydrates a serving. For our purposes, we need to consume beers that come in at that 2.5–3.5 grams per serving sweet spot—a good example of this is Michelob Ultra (2.6 grams carbohydrates—not Michelob Light, which has 11.7 grams carbohydrates). Other choices include Bud Select, Labatt Sterling, Michelob Ultra Amber, Miller Lite, and San Miguel Light.

Mixers For Spirits

When it comes to a choice of mixer for the spirits mentioned above, it is important to avoid fruit juices and obviously sugary soft drinks like cola, lemonade, and "energy" drinks. The best bet is to stick to water, club soda, or a seltzer. If you feel the need for some extra flavor, you can always add a twist of fresh lemon, lime, or orange.

ONE WEEK'S EXAMPLE MENU PLAN

It would be useful to highlight some points about The ONE Diet approach to help individuals maximize the benefits available and prepare for a change in their nutritional intake.

The key to developing new habits is to understand the importance of seeking to enjoy the transition from the old tastes towards new and fresh ways of eating. Enjoyment is vital for the process to be welcomed. To sit and eat something that your taste buds feel repulsion from is ill advised.

Keep in mind that your programming may initially resist the proposed changes on the basis that we have all at some point been indoctrinated about eating "very low-cal" or "low-fat." This, as you will now know, is a fallacy.

Additionally, quality and condition are important to the taste of your nutritional intake. All this adds up to the fact that you will need to become far more discerning in the choice of foods you purchase.

The key ingredients that will need to be curtailed are sugars and grains. Therefore, planning your meals is important, just as having a massive clearout and disposing of all foods that are not in keeping with your best interests.

Taking the time to explore new recipes will increase your interest; visit our site for some great links to other likeminded organizations. You could even discover that you develop a flair for cooking that you never knew you had.

We would suggest that you start the new you on a Sunday. This is so you have sufficient time to prepare and implement your strategy. Prepare your shopping list well in advance and have your meals set out for the week. Do not be alarmed that you will be eating more. It is not how much you are eating; it is all about what you are eating.

Snacks require advanced planning. It is practically useful to carry a few bits that can instantly fulfill your needs far more than the usual kaka burger. The solution is to look for products that are capable of lasting eight to twelve hours outside of a fridge. We have some suggestions, like 100 percent meat salamis, such as the wonderful Negroni Milano salami or French 100 percent sausage salami. Cold cuts of meat are also great options.

Stores are, to some degree, waking up to the need to provide alternatives to sandwiches, so look around and see what fits in with your needs. Avoid the mass-produced, processed variety of meats some corporations produce that contain cheap ingredients as fillers.

Consider having an apple with your favorite cheese. You will be amazed at how full, refreshed, and filled you will feel. Better still, notice how it staves hunger off for far longer that if you were to fill up with some dodgy doughnuts. The doughnuts will leave you feeling hungry again within the hour, and you will experience the nervous, jittery energy that a shot of this sort of kaka will give you, whereas having an apple with some cheese will leave you feeling human again.

Saturday:

Find and dispose of everything that you will not need in your future. Bag it up and take it to a good cause. Remember to check your freezer.

Prepare your list of ingredients and bits that you will need to purchase.

ଔ

Sunday breakfast:
Fried eggs, bacon, tomatoes, and mushrooms

Sunday lunch:
Steak with your favorite healthy vegetables

Sunday dinner:
Portobello mushrooms stuffed with sausage meat, and creamed spinach on the side

ଔ

Monday breakfast:
Fresh fruit with cream

Monday lunch:
Two avocados with plenty of prawns or similar and olive oil

Monday dinner:
Two breasts of chicken, fried or grilled, with melted cheese on top, zucchini/courgettes, broccoli, and string or runner beans

CG

Tuesday breakfast:
Sausages, tomatoes, and plenty of mushrooms cooked in butter

Tuesday lunch:
Tuna and mayonnaise with two avocados

Tuesday dinner:
Baked cod with cauliflower and cheese

CG

Wednesday breakfast:
Fresh fruit salad with cream

Wednesday lunch:
Omelette with salad and tomatoes in olive oil and oregano on the side

Wednesday dinner:
Steak of your choice with steamed vegetables

೫

Thursday breakfast:
A selection of cold meats (salami, etc.) with cheeses

Thursday lunch:
Pickled herrings with beetroot and yoghurt with celery sticks

Thursday dinner:
Prawn and salmon lettuce rolls with a selection of fresh vegetables of your choice

೫

Friday breakfast:

Fresh fruit with yoghurt

Friday lunch:

Grilled tuna steak with asparagus

Friday dinner—treat meal:

Jacket potato royal with your favorite cheese, grated (having a potato is an acceptable treat occasionally; if your goal is weight loss, don't overdo it!)

ಣ

Saturday breakfast:

Scrambled eggs with mushrooms on the side

Saturday lunch:

Minced beef in tomato sauce and broccoli

Saturday dinner:

Roast beef with oven-baked vegetables

ಣ

This example menu is designed to give some idea of the types of foods you can prepare and consume for healthy eating. Have a look at our recipe chapter for more ideas. There are hundreds of cooking combinations you could create. Visit our Web site for great links to amazing recipes where you can also share with others your newfound interest in healthy, tasty eating.

Visit your local fishmonger and let him suggest what fish is in season and incorporate it into your menu. The key is to eat plenty of the right foods and as close to nil of the damaging foods as possible.

Visit your local butcher and explore the different cuts of meat, including offal. Offal is one of the most energy-giving parts of an animal. For instance, discover how many ways you can use lambs' kidneys, because they are full of energy and really tasty, especially on a barbeque. Quality butchers will gladly engage with you once you have shown your interest.

Chapter 11.
The ONE Diet: Finer Points

How Many Meals a Day?

It is worth bearing in mind that many of us are used to consuming some form of energy every couple of hours, or even more often. The body does not require this; in fact, most of us feel hungry and eat again whilst our body is still processing what we last ate.

The fitness, health, and nutrition industries have often made a point over the last couple of decades of telling us to eat a little and often, with up to six small meals a day. Our opinion is that this is unnecessary in terms of both weight loss and general health. The notion that humans have to eat in this way for optimal health and weight loss goals is unfounded. In fact, if we had to eat like this, it is doubtful that our species would have ever survived.

We are not suggesting that you only eat twice a day, although that is a strategy that works very well for some people. The point is not to get caught up in the notion that you have to eat a particular number of times a day, or, for that matter, at set times during the day.

You could eat twice a day or three times a day and healthily lose weight—so long as you are eating the right types of food. Find what works best for you. Relax if scheduling means you have to skip an occasional meal- in fact this may do you some good, as we'll explain when we talk about intermittent fasting.

The Best Quality Meat and Animal Products

Ideally, see if you can source meat that has been pastured (fed grass) or finished on pasture, as opposed to grains. Just as humans have not evolved to eat large quantities of grain, the same is true of most animals. The fat contained in meat sourced from animals fed grain is higher in omega-6 fatty acid—the type we already get far too much of in the West.

This is yet another example of how modern agriculture has altered the food that ends up on our plates. The growing trend of increased awareness amongst health-conscious Americans about this situation has led to an increase in popularity of pastured and pasture-finished meat being labeled as such. In the United States, seek this meat out as best you can.

In the United Kingdom and Europe, the awareness of this situation is somewhat lower and our European readers will perhaps find it more challenging to find meat labeled as pastured. The closest to a solution for our European readers, and what we recommend, is to buy organic meat whenever you can afford to do so. Often the packaging will state what the animal has been fed, and hopefully at least part of its food consumption will have been provided from pasture.

Which Animal Products Are Most Important to Purchase Pastured?

1. Eggs. Buy pastured or organic eggs whenever possible, as the quality of the fat in eggs is greatly determined by the diet of the parent animal.

2. Poultry, pork, and other nonruminant meat. Buy pastured or organic whenever possible, as the quality of the fat in the meat of these animals has a strong correlation with the quality of diet fed to the animal.

3. Fish is another good source of animal protein and fat. When you can, buy wild fish sourced from deep, unpolluted waters. Organic farmed fish are a next-best choice, but avoid regular farmed fish when possible.

4. Beef, lamb, goat, and meat from other ruminant animals contain perhaps the healthiest animal fats that humans consume. The fat contained in ruminant meat that has been pasture fed or pasture finished/organic will be of excellent quality. However, even standard grain-fed ruminant meat will be healthier for us than the first three categories in this list, and so meat from ruminant animals is the least critical to purchase pastured/organic if you are on a budget or have trouble sourcing pastured meat.[1]

Vegetables and Fruits

For some people who are cutting out refined grains and sugars for the first time, they may find fruits, because of their natural sweetness, an attractive option in their new diet. It is important to remember that we need to emphasize vegetables over fruit.

Whilst you can eat as many and as much of our approved vegetables as you want, whenever you want, when reducing weight it is best to exercise some control over fruit consumption to avoid overdoing the fruit sugar fructose. Ideally, eating a maximum of one to two portions of fruit per day will help to ensure you are losing weight at the optimal rate for most people.

Buy seasonal vegetables and fruits that are grown or produced locally whenever possible. Avoid buying commercially grown vegetables and fruits that are of a genetically modified origin.

Dried Fruits

Dried fruits have a far higher ratio of sugar than fresh fruits (fresh fruits contain a high water content, which is missing from dried fruits). This means it is far easier to consume too much sugar by eating dried fruits.

Whilst we recommend steering clear of dried fruits whilst reducing your weight, if eaten occasionally and in moderation, dried fruits may be acceptable.

However, it is always best to view dried fruit as an occasional treat; a portion no larger than a small palmful a couple of times a week is probably fine. Just remember that fresh fruit wins hands down over dried fruit in both weight loss and nutritional terms.

In addition, whenever you can, select organic when purchasing dried fruit (or dry your own), as manufacturers often add sulfur dioxide to commercially dried fruit.

Nuts or Not!

Many people are fine eating raw nuts. However, there are some individuals whose digestive systems may find it a challenge to digest nuts. This is due to elements of the nut that can cause indigestion in some people. If you find this to be the case for you, you can simply avoid nuts, or follow the procedure below to make the nuts more digestible.

Firstly, you will need to soak the raw nuts in salt water overnight. Then take the nuts out of the salt water and rinse them thoroughly. Next, ensure they are dried properly (to avoid mould forming); the quickest way to do this is to put them in the oven on the lowest heat possible until dried.

Facts About Fiber

In addition to the natural sugars contained in plants, cellulose is found in their rigid cell walls. Cellulose is a fiber, which humans are unable to digest. The right amount of fiber in our diet helps with the smooth functioning of our gastrointestinal tract.

Optimally, any fiber in our diets will be derived from vegetables and fruits (as is the case when you follow The ONE Diet) and *not* from the fiber in grains.

When you are following The ONE Diet, you will automatically be getting an appropriate amount of fiber in your diet, primarily from vegetables and secondarily from the fruits you eat.

Despite what many of us have been told in the past about the benefits of fiber, too much dietary fiber (especially fiber derived from grains) actually has a negative effect on our health, as it may enable excess bacteria to flourish in the colon, which can cause discomfort, gas, and even irritable bowel syndrome.

Potatoes, Starchy Root Vegetables and Rice

We have made the point that starch-rich vegetables and rice need to be limited and for some people avoided, during the process of losing weight. In the case of starchy vegetables such as potatoes, you may find a small portion added to a meal has little negative effect on your weight loss progress.

Grains and grain products are simply best avoided from a weight loss and from a health perspective. The one exception to this rule is white rice, a nongluten grain that contains far fewer anti-nutrients and less fiber (remember grain fiber can feed and promote excess bacteria in the colon) than other grains. White rice and products made from rice may be consumed occasionally when the portion size is reasonable.

Once you have attained your goal weight or size, you can fully reintroduce starchy vegetables and white rice into your daily diet, carefully observing any effects they have on your weight/size.

How About Nontoxic Cookware Too?

Now that you're going to be caring more about what you eat and preparing more healthy food, it is best to select your cooking vessels wisely.

The vast majority of nonstick surfaces that cover much cookware available today have been shown to be potentially harmful over the long term. This is another instance where "convenience" and modern manufacturing design are actually inferior to the more traditional and safe cookware available.

So avoid nonstick and/or aluminum cookware, and instead use stainless steel, cast iron, enameled cast iron, or glass cookware whenever possible.

Dealing with the Aftermath of Grain and Sugar Addiction

Putting excess grains and sugars into the human system is a lot like putting very low grade/impure fuel into a car. Yes, the car will go, but it won't work optimally or efficiently, and, over the long term, the engine will get clogged, with the impurities in the fuel putting unnecessary stress on the mechanism, leading to an early breakdown.

The car would have run more smoothly, more efficiently, and have had a longer working lifespan had decent fuel been used in the first place. As it is for the car, it is for the body—put in higher quality food and the body will respond by working more efficiently and effectively, potentially lasting longer. Moreover, in terms of the human body, this means improved general health, less body fat and quite literally more miles per gallon.

When you drastically reduce your consumption of grains, sugars, and the products that contain them, you will quite possibly feel withdrawal symptoms. It works something like this: You get a twinge of hunger and your mind will go to a chocolate bar, a slice of pizza, or bread. To someone new to eating more healthily, this craving may become very strong—the comfort foods of the past are coming back to haunt. The initial positive buzz of refined carbohydrate energy is being remembered.

STOP…what your body is actually telling you is that it needs food. It might need a lot or it might just need a little. Nevertheless, it needs an input of energy fairly soon. It doesn't even need this energy immediately, but your body is reminding you that it will need some food soon.

So take the time to think about what you are going to eat next; do you have it to hand, is it at home or do you need to go shopping to pick it up?

Just thinking through these thoughts will often abate the immediate hunger. You've shown your mind that you have noted your body's needs and will address them soon or at the appropriate time.

If you still feel a little hungry after finishing your meal, we suggest it is best for you to wait ten to twenty minutes or so. Often it takes that amount of time for the food to "land" and your body to tell your mind that it now has been fed, so all is well, and those hunger receptors can be turned off.

I've followed the nutritional plan for four weeks and I'm hardly losing any weight. What specifically do I need to do next?

You are likely one of a very small percentage of individuals whose metabolism is currently particularly sensitive to food intake. Follow the steps below, work your way down the list until you begin to see your weight reduce.

1. Ensure you have completely eliminated from your diet all sugars and foods/drinks containing added sugars and sweeteners, all grains and products made from grains, all vegetable oils, margarines, etc.

2. Consume only one or two portions of berries per day as your total fruit intake.

3. Ensure you have minimized your consumption of; starchy root vegetables (such as potatoes, sweet potatoes, yams, parsnips and cassava), rice and milk. If you have done this already and you are not losing weight, eliminate them completely for now.

4. Experiment with intermittent fasting (see next page).

5. Remember, this five-point plan is to kick-start your metabolism. Once your weight is starting to drop consistently, you can experiment with

reintroducing some acceptable carbohydrates like starchy vegetables and more fruits back into your diet, observing the effect this has on your weight loss. If you continue to lose one or two pounds of weight per week or your body measurements are decreasing, you are eating the right amount for you.

Intermittent Fasting—The Simplest Guide

Intermittent fasting can boost weight loss results for those at a sticking point. Intermittent fasting simply means going for a little longer between meals than you usually would.

Intermittent fasting has been shown to effectively decrease blood pressure, reduce oxidative damage to DNA, lipids, and protein, and improve insulin sensitivity and glucose uptake.

Four slightly differing approaches to intermittent fasting:

—Skip breakfast altogether.

—Every now and then, we can just randomly decide to skip one of our regular planned meals during a day.

—We may deliberately limit ourselves to just two planned meals on a particular day—one in the morning and one in the afternoon or evening—and no eating on that day outside of the two meals.

—We can have a pre-planned fast for eighteen hours straight through.

When intermittent fasting, avoid overeating in the periods before or after the fast; the aim is to eat what you need, not more to make up for what you haven't had or won't be having over the coming hours.

Changing the Eating Habits of a Lifetime

Imagine that you have learned to type with two fingers. You have mastered typing fast with your two index fingers, but one day you discover that other people can type much faster than you can. You realize that you too could type faster if you changed your way of typing.

It appears that with two fingers you may reach a speed of sixty words a minute. However, with all your fingers you could double that speed. Initially you may be eager to switch typing styles and experience a feeling of excitement when you think about it.

Here we reach a dichotomy. In order to develop a faster typing style, we will need to stop using two fingers and start using all of them. The difficulty arises when we realize that our typing has slowed down considerably. Where you were typing sixty words per minute, now you are down to twenty-five words a minute. The temptation is to switch back to typing as you have in the past. Correct persistence is required if you are to successfully make the transition.

The temptation to go back to using two fingers is compelling. There could be frustration and anger developing. There could be embarrassment that you have to slow down and that others in the office will see that you are fumbling with the keyboard and making several errors.

Concentration will need to be developed in order to speed up. You will, in a matter of days, notice that your speed is improving and that you are almost up to your old speed, and day by day you are increasing that speed.

Then the day arrives that you break your previous record and exceed sixty words a minute. Each day there is an improvement until you reach your potentiality. Suddenly you realize that two things have occurred. The first is that you are typing faster than you have ever typed in the past. The second is that you no longer need to be focused on your typing technique. The whole process has become automated.

With the help of this book, we anticipate that initially there may be some resistance to changing your dietary consideration. The probability is that your existing patterns will seek to be satisfied and will fight for continuity, on the basis that it is what our mind has become accustomed to and what it knows. However, just as in the typing example above, with correct persistence you will be able to win at weight loss.

Chapter 12.
Boost Your Body with the Best Exercise

"When diet and exercise are properly understood...gone will be the days of weighing food, counting calories, and plodding along on the treadmill for hours. When you eat a proper diet, and partake of high-intensity exercise, you set into motion a vicious positive cycle that makes the body you desire easy to achieve."

Doug McGuff, MD

The Role of Exercise in Fat Loss

The role of exercise in fat loss is often overstated, yet it is important when done correctly. The biggest misunderstanding made by many people is the belief that low or medium intensity exercise such as "aerobics" or "cardiovascular exercise" can burn off plenty of calories.

Although it is beyond the scope of this book to discuss the subject of exercise in its entirety, it is worth our while to cover the fundamentals of exercise as it relates to weight loss and well-being. For those who wish to understand exercise fully, we highly recommend reading *Body by Science*, written by Doug McGuff, MD, and John Little.

There is one form of exercise that easily wins when it comes to improving metabolism, building healthy lean tissue, and driving our bodies to "burn" off stored fat. The form of exercise we are talking of is high intensity strength training.

When applied correctly, high intensity strength training need be performed only once or twice a week for a maximum of twenty minutes per session.

The Effects of High Intensity Strength Training on Weight Loss and Hunger

High intensity strength training has a unique effect on our bodies when it comes to losing weight that no other form of exercise or activity can match. When we perform a high intensity strength training workout, we kick into action a cascade of beneficial metabolic effects.

Initially there is a release of adrenaline, which then requires the body to utilize large amounts of glycogen (stored energy) out of our muscles. This has the effect of emptying our muscles of their excess glucose, which will need to be replaced.

To do this, our bodies will restore the insulin receptors on the muscle surface; levels of glucose in our blood stream then drop. Following this hormone-sensitive lipase begins to enable the release of our own stored body fat to use as an immediate energy source. This is actually what happens when you "burn" off fat.

There is another huge benefit to the fact that your body is now using its own supplies of stored fat to create energy, and that is, hunger levels actually decrease.

When you eat and exercise in the way we recommend, you will be burning off your body fat and your hunger levels will decrease. When you do feel hungry, it will be noticeable as a subtle signal to think about getting some food soon, rather than, "Oh my goodness, I've got to have something sugary right now!"

You will notice that when you follow our advice, even when you do feel that gentle sensation of hunger, if you ignore it for five or ten minutes it will fade, and you won't notice it again for a while.

Plus, you will only feel hungry when your body cannot get enough energy from using its own fat stores for its immediate needs. In this scenario, your body is essentially burning off its own fat stores as fast as it possibly and healthily can.

By combining our healthy, natural diet with a once- or twice-a-week, twenty-minute, high intensity strengthening program, you are giving your body the metabolic advantage that is your birthright and you will be maximizing your personal genetic potential to look, feel, and be the best that you can, no matter what your current size or age.

High intensity strength training creates a further benefit for our weight loss goals and that is our muscles will be able to store more glycogen. This means even if we do occasionally eat too much, less of that food energy will be converted into fat as our muscles will be able to store more of the glucose as glycogen.

High intensity strength training also increases levels of the hormone adiponectin. Adiponectin can help to combat major health issues, including coronary artery and cerebral artery disease and fattening of the liver, and simultaneously improves both insulin sensitivity and triglyceride (fat) metabolism.

"Resistance exercise does increase REE (resting energy expenditure) and adiponectin in an intensity-dependent manner…. It appears that resistance exercise may represent an effective approach for weight management and metabolic control."[1]

You'll notice that the research above also mentions that high intensity strength training increases resting energy expenditure, which is another massive bonus for those of us looking to reduce our weight.

What this means is that after you've finished your twenty-minute workout, your body is consuming elevated amounts of energy. So long as you're not overeating the wrong types of food, you'll have stimulated the body to "burn" off its own fat even when you're resting or just carrying out your normal daily activities, long after the workout has finished.

This particular piece of research showed that resting energy expenditure remained elevated for forty-eight hours after the workout. This is even before your body has synthesized new lean tissue (muscle) as a result of the workout, which will then lead to an even greater fat-burning effect over the rest of the week till your next workout. Now that really is a great return on investment for your twenty minutes spent working out once or twice a week.

Resistance exercise also increases lipolysis (fat burning) during and after the workout by stimulating the release of the hormones epinephrine, norepinephrine, and growth hormone. One study showed that fat oxidation was 105 percent higher after resistance training than in the control group.[2]

The Core Benefits of High Intensity Strength Training

- Burns calories and turns our bodies into more efficient fat-burning machines by raising our metabolic rate

- Helps normalize body fat levels and improves our physical appearance—the sexy, lean, and toned look

- Improves health issues, including blood pressure, diabetes, heart disease, and cholesterol levels

- Improves heart function and cardiovascular condition

- Strengthens and "tones" the muscles

- Increases our physical energy levels

- Protects our joints

- Improves our ability to perform most other physical activities

Your High Intensity Workout

We recommend that everybody start out with a workout known as the "Big Five," as suggested by Doug McGuff, MD, and John Little in *Body by Science*, which consists of the following exercises performed on good quality weight machines:

1) Seated row

2) Chest press

3) Pulldown

4) Overhead press

5) Leg press

These five exercises efficiently and effectively work all the major muscles of the body including the postural muscles like the abdominals.

You will perform all the exercises in a smooth and controlled manner. This means performing the exercises slowly, not rushing through the movements. Your speed of movement will be around five seconds up and five seconds down, or slower. This deliberate speed of movement eliminates momentum from the exercises, ensuring that your muscles do all the work.

The aim is to do each exercise until the targeted musculature is fatigued and you can no longer move the resistance. Find a weight for each exercise in your initial workout that allows you to perform the movement for between forty-five seconds and two minutes. For example, on your first workout, you may manage to get these times with an appropriate weight for you on each exercise:

Seated row—ninety-five seconds seconds

Chest press—eighty-eight seconds

Pulldown—ninety seconds

Overhead press—seventy-three seconds

Leg press—ninety-eight seconds

You are only to perform one single "set" of each exercise that ideally lasts somewhere between forty-five seconds and two minutes.

Use a stopwatch to record your times for each exercise and note them down immediately—this way, you can track your progress from workout to workout. Even a couple of seconds' increase in each movement from one session to the next shows improvement in your body. Once you can perform an exercise at a given weight for longer than two minutes that is a sign to increase the weight used on that exercise at your next scheduled workout.

You may take a brief rest break between each exercise of up to a minute, but once you've started an exercise, continue that particular exercise until physically you cannot perform another repetition with good technique. Do not stop for a rest, then start the same exercise again—once you have started the stopwatch, you keep going on that exercise until you can do no more; stop the stopwatch, record your time, then move onto the next movement.

You will be performing this workout once or twice a week, leaving a minimum of four days between workouts. So if you perform your first workout on a Monday the earliest you will perform your next workout is Friday—or you could just wait until the following Monday.

The recovery time between workouts is where your body will actually be making the positive changes the workout has stimulated, so it is important that you leave at least four days between workouts. Working out more frequently will ultimately stymie your progress.

To learn more about this type of exercise and to view technique videos of each exercise and complete workouts visit Dr. McGuff's Web site, www.bodybyscience.net. You can find a personal trainer or gym in your area that specializes in high intensity training, by going to the Directory page on that Web site.

Are You Sure I Don't Need to Do More Exercise?

Please bear in mind that excess exercise can halt weight loss progress. Remember that using low or medium intensity exercise to burn off calories is extremely inefficient (it takes a heck of a lot of activity to burn off a relatively small number of calories), and too much exercise stimulates unnecessary hunger.

Many people fall into the trap of believing that because they exercised for an hour, they can treat themselves to a sweet "treat." An hour on the treadmill may cause 250 calories more to be metabolized than if you were at rest. At the same time, a well-known regular, individual-size chocolate, nougat, and caramel bar contains 280 calories. So even before you take into account the massive 42.6 grams of carbohydrate in the supersweet chocolate bar, if you run for an hour on the treadmill, then eat one of these bars, you've already consumed more calories than you used by running on the treadmill.

We also need to consider the fact that low or medium intensity activity (e.g., jogging, running, aerobics, etc.) carried out for durations like our example of the hour on the treadmill will likely result in a loss of muscle tissue over time due to overuse atrophy. It's usually quite a slow process, but over the course of a year, a person could lose around four pounds of muscle tissue from this type of training.

Loss of muscle tissue, of course, means a lowered metabolic rate, which means the body burns or uses fewer calories twenty-four hours a day. This will lead to more fat storage—it's that vicious cycle again! Keep this important point in mind: a person who believes exercise can make up for poor dietary habits and excessive carbohydrate consumption is fighting a losing battle.

You've now been introduced to an exercise method that will maximally stimulate fat loss and optimize metabolically important lean tissue, a method that you can perform in just twenty minutes once or twice a week. Do you need to do anything else?

The short answer is no! You will have covered all the health and weight loss benefits that can be derived from exercise in your high intensity strength training sessions. You will have achieved all those benefits in an efficient, effective, and safe manner.

There is no need to spend hours per week at the gym, in an aerobics class, pounding the streets running, on the treadmill, elliptical trainer, vibrating machine, indoor rower, or any other type of equipment. In fact, doing too much medium intensity exercise can not only slow or even halt your weight loss progress but it also puts your joints under too much repetitive strain that may lead to long-term health issues.

What we do highly recommend in addition to high intensity strength training is *recreation*. What we mean by recreation is physical activities you engage in for sheer pleasure.

Walking or, Even Better, Strolling

We are big fans of walking. Just getting outside for a stroll or even a hike when you have the time gets your body moving in a very gentle and natural way. It will also enable you to get some fresh air and some very beneficial sunshine (think vitamin D production).

We're not talking about speed walking or anything like that; we're talking about strolling, ambling along, enjoying the sights and sounds, taking some time for yourself to recharge your batteries and to get the blood gently flowing. If you can get outside for a daily walk of between ten minutes and an hour, or several short walks throughout the day/evening, we guarantee you'll feel good. We recommend that everyone take at least a short walk every day.

The Benefits of Daily Walking

- Improves your immune system

- Improves mood

- Improves quality of life

- Improves sense of well-being

- Relieves stress

- Increases blood and oxygen flow throughout the body, including the brain

- Provides an opportunity to reflect and ruminate

- Is low impact on your joints

Sports

Some people may enjoy participating in a recreational sport, anything from squash or tennis to an informal game of football in the park. So long as *you* enjoy it and don't overdo it, or push yourself too hard or too often, it will add benefit to your life. Remember, these are not activities you have to do. Only get involved in a sport if you enjoy it and it is pleasurable for you.

A word of caution:

For some people, when they begin to make lifestyle changes, they can go over the top and think if some exercise is good, then more must be better. Those people may spend a lot of money on an expensive piece of exercise equipment or gym membership that they use for a couple of weeks and then forget about. Or, they may become obsessed by exercise and drive themselves to over exercise nearly every day until they burn out.

Remember, healthy lifestyle choices add to your life rather than take away from it, giving you more energy on balance rather than depleting your reserves. Exercise is similar to food, in that too much of it is ultimately as bad for us as too little. Avoid running your body into the ground through obsessively over exercising.

Perhaps you'd enjoy dancing more. Joining a local salsa class or any other style of dancing can be a lot of fun, plus you'll have some personal interaction—and for those of you who are single, you may even meet someone you'd enjoy dating!

Of course, there are other possibilities, too, and they don't need to be overly physical. Many people derive benefit from a weekly or monthly massage or learning to relax and switch off through meditation.

Explore these and other options and find what works best to enhance your life.

Chapter 13.
Super Successful Strategies

Select one of the strategies suggested below and work through it. Once you feel you have mastered it, you may select another strategy to work on. Avoid trying to do more than one strategy at a time.

Needs and Wants

Whilst conflicts exist between what we need and what we want, there will be a struggle to contain the "fat fight." It is therefore important to create an atmosphere of understanding, cooperation, and tolerance for both if we are to accomplish our objectives.

This strategy requires that we acknowledge the current state of our needs and our wants. It requires that we step out of our emotions and take the stance similar to that of a relationship counselor.

We simply stand between the two elements "without taking either side" and just explore what the current views are from both our needs and wants as if they are two separate parts of ourselves.

By treating needs and wants as if they are two separate entities, we are more able to understand each part's viewpoint better. It is only when we understand the driving force behind our actions that we can be in a place to seek and find a better solution that satisfies our needs and wants.

The key to this strategy is simple: do not take either side. It is not about who is right and who is wrong; it is about understanding each side's position and showing compassion with each. It is about befriending both needs and wants. It is about being able to be a good friend to both if we are to avoid a yo-yo relationship where each side has thoughtless control and abuses the other.

The Strategy

Make approximately thirty minutes available without being disturbed (no phones, TV, etc.) and find a comfortable chair. Perhaps sit with a pad and pen nearby in case you need to make notes, and imagine to your right and left each part preparing their position to present to you.

Internally communicate with each part separately and give enough time for each to tell you their story. In some cases, it may sound like history where the story is mostly about what they had missed out on. In some instances it may be, that you will be informed of how they had been denied sweets through their life, or that they were treated badly and that this is a kind of payback for those years.

Make notes where you need to. Get as true and meaningful an understanding of the drivers behind the behaviors of both your "needs" and "wants." Be caring and sincere about their respective perspectives.

Remember, it is not about who is right and who is wrong; it is more about hearing what their conflict is about. It may be that "needs" has the expectation of being superfit with the stunningly toned body of a sixteen-year-old cheerleader. Okay, so that is what is desired and sought. The likelihood of that happening we know to be unrealistic, but just hear what their perspective is and how they have reasoned it out.

There is no right or wrong; there just "is." It is just the state of affairs, and this is a report of the state of the union between "needs and wants." Think about each perspective and review the information received. Understand that there may be many truths and that they exist within you.

By following this process, we are finally getting to grips with the victims in this tragedy. Both "needs" and "wants" have a right to what they perceive as being their prerogative and drive. The erroneous thoughts, once brought to light, will impact on our understanding and therefore our future action.

It is anticipated that by understanding the drivers, a change in direction will ensue. Keep in mind that it may be that the original expectations were unrealistic. It may be that both "needs and wants" will learn about each other and respect each other's perspective. It is highly likely that the newfound information contained within this book will have changed your perspective in any event.

Consensus is where we seek a point of agreement, unlike compromise, where both parties in a negotiation have to give up something. When we realize we are in the midst of a futile war, where no progress can be made and the only thing that happens is the destruction of our resources, we can begin to see that carrying on is futile.

Perhaps each part may realize that the other is struggling and that at the end there will be two losers and ultimately you all lose. If that is where consensus is, then great progress has been made. Disease and discomfort will be the final outcome if we continue doing what we have always done.

By allowing expression of needs and wants, we might discover reasons for maintaining our size and shape that we had not previously acknowledged. The drivers that motivated this perspective may result in a new perspective being developed that includes needs and wants working in harmony.

Have a go and discover what needs to happen for you to be at peace with your size and weight.

Self-Awareness

As mentioned previously, we need to be aware of what we look like in order to realize what we need to do to correct the situation. In some instances, we might be shocked at realizing the situation is worse than we have imagined.

This strategy will help bring about new motivation where needed or calm the mind where it had become overly desperate. It requires that a clear and accurate picture of your body shape and size is represented to your mind anew.

The image we hold of ourselves tends to be a snapshot of that we have attached to, which rarely gets challenged. It may be that we have seen an image of ourselves in a picture or a video and stuck with it.

This can be evidenced when we meet up with friends who we have not seen in years and are surprised at how much they have changed. Only then do we stop and have another look at how we have aged and "grown."

It is as though a new perspective was hoisted upon us and woke us up to a realization that we were previously oblivious to. We do age and we do change shape. Often we need this type of jolt to get into action.

We may see an old friend and discover that we had not realized just how much they consumed at a dinner. It may be that we are the ones that seem to go crazy at the restaurant, ordering enough for three. Our awareness may bring us to the realization that in fact we overconsume in comparison to someone who is able to maintain a healthier body than ours.

The Strategy

Make the necessary time available to ensure that you are able to bring about the actions required. Using a digital camera (often found on mobile phones), in your private space, start to take pictures of yourself from as many angles as possible.

Start with full body shots from front and back. A timer may be appropriate to take the photograph, unless you have a partner who is helping to facilitate your change program. Take shots of side views, back views, standing, sitting, slouching, etc., and, once collected, inspect the perspectives as an observer. Avoid becoming emotionally involved.

Now have a look at each photograph. Does it fit in with what you thought you looked like? Is it better, is it worse or is it as you thought? Now just consider, with the knowledge you have, what has caused your body to become as you see it. Is it lack of awareness, is it denial, is it lack of information, is it lack of realization? Explore and sense what seems to be the case for you. It could be a combination of things.

Next, decide if you want to do anything about this. If so, decide what you can do with the resources you have. Start small and be consistent. It is pointless becoming desperate about the situation. This will only instill fear and result in more anxiety being created, thereby defeating the object.

Select a plan from the suggestions in this book and quietly get on with what needs to happen to get you to the place where, when you take the time to look at yourself properly again, you can see a difference occurring. Avoid seeking perfection, as you will discover; unless you are suffering from narcissism, there is no such thing as perfection or imperfection. Therefore, you are evolving into a new you every day.

Let at least a month go by before you start the process again.

Picture the Outcome

In accordance with the way our mind operates, the clearer the outcome we seek, the more likely our mind will "will" us there. Remember that what we dwell upon becomes the focus of our attention. So, it would be prudent to avoid being focused on what we do not want. It makes more sense to have an image of what we do want to look like.

The Strategy

If you have a photograph of yourself looking close to how you want to shape up to be, then have that image on your computer screen or somewhere like the fridge door. Keep the image of the shape you are aspiring to reach foremost in your mind.

In the event that you are unable to find such an image, look in a magazine for a photograph of the shape you seek to be that does not show the facial features of the person in the photograph. It is an image of the shape you seek, no more than that.

Keep in mind that your mind is not stupid, and having an image of a person that is not your body type will do nothing but aggravate the situation. Keeping it real keeps it alive.

Best Friend

Some people may need to have external support. This in many ways is why so many join groups and organizations that specialize in weight control. There are compelling reasons in being with a group.

There is a camaraderie that develops in a group that would otherwise not exist for a person doing this on his or her own. There is a pressure to please your facilitator. There is also useful information that individuals share in a group that can give fresh ideas and can inspire those who have struggled. It is a great place to be encouraged and celebrated when someone accomplishes a goal.

For some people it is important to have this level of support, and, where possible, we would encourage support for those that feel that they cannot do this on their own. Better to have support than to suffer in silence.

In the event that you cannot cope with the whole group thing, you might find that enlisting the help of a very close and supportive friend brings you just what you need in terms of support—a little like having a sponsor, who will be there at times when you just need to let off some steam.

Remember, this will be a short dependence, as we would estimate that within a month or two, you will have completely changed your eating habits. You might find that you accomplish more with having someone to talk to.

The Strategy

Enlist the help of someone who you consider dependable and nonjudgmental. Explain the task that you have set yourself and that you will need supporting for a short time. This will involve the person committing to be there for you in an emergency and agreeing that you will contact him or her once per week with your progress.

Explain that it will not involve him or her giving you any nutritional information and that he or she will not have to do anything whatsoever other than talk with you in the event you have the need to let off some steam.

From your part, you will need to commit to calling the person once per week with your progress report, no matter how you are progressing. Good weeks and not-so-good weeks, you still need to call. You have made a contract with someone by enlisting his or her support, so you will need to honor your side of the deal.

In an ideal situation, it would be handy if it were not someone you see every day, though this would not be unmanageable. Someone perhaps who you know and now lives some distance away.

Having the support does not mean that you become unreasonable and call any time of day, no matter how you might be feeling. Respect for others extends respect to you. So be considerate, and should they be unable for whatever reason to continue, just accept that it is in your best interest and ensure that closure is appropriate.

Criticism and Self-Image

All criticism converts to become self-criticism. When you are comparing other people's size detrimentally, you are then focused on the negative aspects of weight loss. Remind yourself that what you focus on and what you allow yourself to dwell upon is what your mind perceives you as being and wanting.

If the objective is to make yourself feel better by observing another person's misfortune, you are going about it in the most destructive way possible. You will either become the object of ridicule/comparison, or you will live in the fear of being the same as the very person you are being critical of.

It is really simple: just accept that everyone is doing the best he or she knows to do. Not making a judgment simply requires that you can observe, yet have no opinion about him or her. Others are simply humans being. Accept that you may not know what caused that person to be as they are and just move on.

When it comes to self-criticism, you will need to be vigilant. The mind is a "yes" mechanism. Whatever we say to ourselves is met with a "yes" response. If you say, "I am so fat," the mind acts by accepting this literally. If you were to say, "This is difficult," your mind responds with a "yes" and then ensures that it makes it so.

Have no doubt of the importance of the words you are using about yourself and when you speak of yourself and others. The mind does not differentiate between saying things about others and saying things about ourselves. What matters, and can often be evident in the intimation of your tonality, is your intention.

Let's explore what happens when something negative is said. If you were to say, "She's a fat cow," the mind seeks to extract meaning. What is your point? So what? Which means what?

If what you mean is that she is "in some way ugly," then it is likely that you also, on some level and at certain times, look at yourself in some way as being ugly, or at the very least worry that you might be seen as "fat and ugly."

In essence, it is all about projection. Whatever you say of others is simply a projection of yourself. You are talking about yourself through another. The key is to be aware of such negative statements.

Be conscious of your intention. Is it that if you can see someone else as being worse than you are, that makes you feel temporarily better? If it is so, then you will need to understand that this type of thinking leads to self-deception and makes the process of weight loss for you fraught with dangers.

The Strategy

Keep your thoughts "good." You know when you are being good; there is a kindness about you. You are not judging anyone; you are simply allowing others to be.

If you have nothing nice to say about another human being, then say or think nothing. Just observe, accept, and move on. The less attention you give to where you do not want to be going, the quicker you get to where you want to be.

Initially, you might discover that you have been involved unknowingly in serious self-sabotage through negative projections. Each time you notice yourself saying something negative about another person, correct the situation by finding three positive things to say about them.

Let's suppose that you see someone who is not the size you want to be, and you make a negative statement about her: "She is stuffing her face like a pig, so gross." The implication of disgust is somewhat obvious. Correct this immediately by finding or imagining three positive things about her.

This could be "She has a great eye for color," "She looks after her hair," and "She is very polite to people around her." Should your mind start again, then you will need to find yet another three things. Your mind will soon learn who the boss is. Stamp your authority; show your mind what will happen from now on.

The outcome over a relatively short period will be a calmness that you notice only when you stop to notice how much more at peace your mind is without the constant critic.

Self-Care Development

Self-care is not something that comes naturally to us. It does happen when parents have taken the time and the right approach to instill values that include self-care. Here we are not talking about the "remember to brush your teeth" hygiene care; we are talking about a self-care that includes the care of our body above and beyond hygiene.

Think about the amount of time we spend on shopping for clothing, computers, the Internet, telephones, gossip and newsmongering, bijou items, makeup, our children's and pets' welfare, the time we spend in gyms and solariums and with the infernal television and the like.

The community face we project and maintain, as well as keeping up with the neighborhood appearance, is mostly about care of perceived image and things that make us into someone we want the world to see us as being.

What goes on internally and the comfort level of our body may not get a look in. It is almost as if we do not really matter. We are just coasting along in a state of indifference about our well-being.

Is it not pitiful that we have simply not been taught to care about our well-being on a nutritional level? Is it not strange that in schools we are not taught to think about how to maintain our being? We are not taught how to consume healthy foods that enhance and improve the quality of our own physical, mental, and emotional experience.

The Strategy

Set aside about five minutes per day for approximately a month. Select an area of your nutritional or physical life and explore if you are being as aware and as caring as you need to be. For example, you might start by noting what vegetables are in season. Perhaps do some research and discover what vegetables are grown locally. You might seek out where a local farm is located.

On a different day, you might spend some time considering different muscles in your body, and just ponder on what you can do to make life more comfortable for them. Better nutrition, some movements that might help them develop more strength for you.

Stop, think, and act in your body's interest.

Common Sense

It is obvious that if you go out shopping without knowing what you want, you are opening yourself up to the probability of being influenced by whatever is around you. You will be at the mercy of the clever advertising, as well as being influenced by the smell of the bakery department and the ready-to-take-home meals.

Common sense implies that we are thoughtful, logical, have considered many aspects of any given situation, and have selected the best solution by considering the consequences of our choice.

It is therefore prudent to think through your actions when considering your nutrition. If you put yourself at risk, you are likely to increase the possibility of compromising yourself.

There are several ways of minimizing the risks, and here we list a few of the most obvious.

Avoid food shopping when hungry

Hunger pangs are a very powerful driver. All we can see suddenly becomes a taste to desire. Often, reasoning is lost as instinct overrides all rational thoughts.

List your needs and wants for the week

By following a process that you have created yourself, you are far less likely to be persuaded by others to buy something you did not set out to purchase. Lists seriously minimize the chances of being distracted. A key to it is to work out the cost of your shopping on the first occasion and take enough cash to cover the cost.

Lists make it clear as to what is permissible and what is not. They are a reminder of your intention and serve to keep you on track. Use a simple phrase such as *"If it's not on the list, it doesn't exist."*

Use online shopping

When possible, shop online if you find there is less temptation for you to pick up unhealthy items. Never subscribe to food sites that will bombard you with their daily offers. Resist being the hamster in the cage that will be subjected to other people's will.

Avoid free tasters

Avoid "taste this, it's free" type of offers. There is a reason behind any company wanting you to taste its product. It wants you to buy it. Stop, think, and act in your best interest.

Avoid free money-back offers

"If you do not like it, we will give you your money back." By tasting it, you open your mind to the possibility of reasoning a way of justifying the purchase. Avoid the temptation.

Only store what you eat for the week

Never keep food in your home that you know to be damaging your system. Stop the "it's just in case someone pops round" or "sometimes the kids bring their friends." Any excuse is just that, an excuse to slip back. If you have anything in your home that is nutritionally damaging, then remember it's a risk.

Avoid judging others

It can be just as damaging to sit in judgment of others' habits, as it is to scold yourself for minor misdemeanors. The less time spent dwelling on negative elements, the better. Focus on the goodness around.

Resist temptation

Become the best carer you can be to yourself. Others may not fully understand what you have to do to get yourself healthy. Learn to say "thank you…no."

Use positive humor

Humor can successfully disrupt negative and unwanted emotions. It is by far more beneficial to laugh at the tactics used by the corporations than to get angry. If you find yourself attaching to an advert, stop and look at it from an aspect that allows you to have a laugh. When you are caught out by some sales advertising, stop, observe, and think, "How desperate those people are."

Avoid arguments

There is no mileage in getting into an argument with those around you that persist in maintaining their old patterns. The trap that they are in no longer serves you, and, therefore, engaging in argument—"I am right—you are wrong"—simply keeps you unnecessarily connected to the negative elements of your food intake. Be pleased that others have something that works for them.

Avoid processed foods

Now that you have the facts about food that has been tampered with, as best you can avoid purchasing processed foods. Occasionally it may be unavoidable. Let that be the exception, and accept that in the main you can avoid it.

Use rituals to your benefit

Often, for many, having a ritual can have a very beneficial effect. Set time aside to engage in a process that focuses your attention upon an act. Rituals help us to expand our awareness of a subject matter and encourage an interest in a specific topic.

If you create a ritual, such as when shopping you only buy what is on the list, you will, over a short period, learn to be more thoughtful and consequently more selective about your purchases. Another type of ritual is to spend a few minutes every morning, perhaps when you are in the bathroom, planning your nutritional intake for the day.

The benefit of showing your mind what and when you will eat seriously helps to avoid fears that would otherwise be present around food.

Make contempt your stop sign

Contempt serves as a stop sign in the mind. What we show contempt towards; we are highlighting our disinterest about. This is more for items and things that we would otherwise have bought. We might see a "cat and mouse" ice cream that we would have otherwise been enticed by. Now we show contempt toward it. These items have been partially responsible for the extra fat we are carrying.

If you are uncertain about contempt, study someone who is good at it. Differentiate between being cynical and being contemptuous. The cynic is getting off on it; the contemptuous is disgusted by it.

Never jest about your size

Never, ever joke about your size. Remember that more often than not, your mind cannot tell the difference. Self-made comments such as "Guys like big girls" or "Big is beautiful" may not be in your best interest—not unless you want your mind to give you more of the same. In some ways, you are inviting a dangerous possibility.

The past is no longer the present

Avoid conversations about what you used to do. Talk more about what are you doing now and how you are doing it. Talk about what you have accomplished and how much better things are now that you have developed your style of weight loss. Re-imprinting the past can be dangerous and in most cases needs to be avoided. Stay focused on your accomplishments, even if they appear small at times.

Chapter 14.
In Conclusion

Changes in perception of food, nutrition, and diet are essential to bringing about physical and psychological transformation for our well-being.

The ONE Diet covers the affects of advertising, marketing, and ploys used by the food and diet industries to directly or indirectly, covertly or overtly, breach our defense mechanism so as to render us incapable of tending to our nutritional needs healthily.

With the explosion of television advertising, video, billboards, social media groups, and affiliate programs, more and more opportunities have been created to exploit and control us. We are mostly unaware of the vulnerable position we have been left in.

The quality of our food has been eroded. In many cases the "food" we eat has been modified in such ways that it is damaging to our organism. Most mass-produced foods have been processed to the degree of bearing little resemblance to healthy, natural produce.

Furthermore, the ingredients that dominate the typical modern Western diet are both the cheapest to produce and the most damaging to our health. This includes cereal grains, sugars and sweeteners, plant oils and hydrogenated fats.

The crux of the problem of obesity and weight gain in today's world lies in the dramatic increase in the consumption of refined carbohydrates.

The misconceptions surrounding healthy as to opposed to unhealthy fats is clarified as we understand that all hydrogenated oils and most vegetable and plant oils are unhealthy and can severely damage the system. Conversely, eating natural saturated fats present in real foods is vital and fundamental to human existence.

The mind's ability to continue doing what it has always done, once it has been programmed to do so, is both genius and sometimes a dance with the devil. Our ability to create repetitive programs can leave us trapped in habits that are damaging to our very existence. Unless we stop and challenge the basis for our eating regimes, we will remain trapped in old behaviors.

Psychological considerations have been thoroughly explored to give insight as to how events in our childhood can severely impact our self-image and beliefs about our abilities. Breaking patterns is the challenge that this book offers. Reviewing self-image and beliefs about who we are and what our life is about needs to come to the forefront of our daily activities for a while.

All the research included in *The ONE Diet* has been thoroughly explored for those who have a need to get to the truth. The scientific information, in a clear and digestible format, evidences the facts for the discerning reader. In essence, we are now aware that what we had been told in the past about nutrition was a carefully crafted illusion, and the facts speak for themselves.

Just as you would not go to a magician to lose weight, we would not expect anyone with half a brain to think that by taking a miracle pill we are going to alter our nutritional needs. The facts speak for themselves, and there are no alternatives and no exceptions to eating well. Just eat natural foods that have not been tampered with from the lists provided, and the rest is a walk in the park.

Setting realistic goals is vital to developing a healthy body, as is developing a respectful attitude towards yourself and others who are in a similar place. Remember that where you focus your attention is where you are heading. Sitting in judgment of others has been proven to be damaging to oneself. If you cannot be nice to others or to yourself, then have no opinion. Just get on with what you are doing and treat it as a process. At best, you can teach your mind great things by seeing yourself and others in a better light. Learning to be kind and considerate will further enhance your experience of living.

Simply use *The ONE Diet* and the included exercises to achieve your desired weight. Resources are included to make the transition more manageable. The use of a food dairy and selected strategies all go some way to helping make the process accomplishable and therefore more likely to lead to success.

We wish you the very best and would love to hear of your successes on our Web site, www.theonediet.com.

Chapter 15.
Recipes

STEAK

Beef steaks

Steak is perhaps the most rewarding of foods from a nutritional perspective. Ideally, the meat would be pasture raised and hung for up to twenty-one days.

The sizes vary from around 3 inches or 7 centimeters for an average fillet steak to 7 inches or 16 centimeters for a small T-bone steak.

Preparation

A common error is to cook the steak straight from the fridge. We would recommend that it be left at room temperature to relax for an hour or more. The local temperature needs to be considered. We tend to take the meat out in the morning for grilling or pan frying on the same evening.

During relaxing time, you can season with a mix of dried lemon pepper and a teaspoon of teriyaki sauce rubbed lightly on both sides.

The cuts of beef vary considerably in tenderness and texture. The best cut is probably **fillet** steak, also known as

tenderloin steak, which tends to be a more expensive cut. The cuts can vary in size; we would recommend 9 ounce or 200- to 250-gram portions.

Rib-eye steaks are recognizable by the additional natural fat content layered in the meat. A lovely way to prepare them during their relaxing stage is to cut into the fat with a small, sharp knife and add some wasabi sauce, into the cut. About a level teaspoon per steak with seasoning will work wonderfully. In terms of size, a good portion would be about 9–14 ounces or 250–400 grams.

T-bone steak is another great cut which is also favored by meat lovers. It is characterized by the T-shaped vertebrae and large muscle. In addition to the tenderness of the meat, there is also the added flavor of the bone, which adds to tenderness of the meat. The portion size would be about 12 ounces or 350 grams upwards.

Porterhouse steak is similar to the T-bone, though the muscle is slightly larger and has no bone.

Sirloin steak is also boneless and as tender as porterhouse.

Cooking

There is a variety of methods for cooking steaks, ranging from pan-frying to oven roasting. We would recommend pan-frying.

Melt a small amount of ghee or butter in a heavy-based pan. Place the steak in the pan and cook uncovered.

Generally, and dependent on personal preference, we would recommend only turning the meat over once during cooking to avoiding overly drying the steak. The point is to sear the meat so as it seals in the flavor.

Cooking time varies from cut to cut, and as a rule of thumb, we would suggest for a medium steak that is cooked through but left slightly pink, about 1 minute per 3.5 ounces or 100 grams.

Adding strong flavors can detract from the meat's natural flavors, so go sparingly with any additions. We might suggest adding butter and a touch of garlic or very mild onion during the heating of the pan.

When broiling steak, very lightly coat the meat cut with a little ghee and seasoning, then place on a rack until it has reached your desired finish.

Cooking in the oven can produce a great result if the oven is able to reach around 480°F or 250°C. Coat the meat in the usual way and place on a rack at the top of the oven. With cuts like ribeye, if possible, stand on the narrow side to allow for a more balanced heat.

After removing meat from the oven, allow a few minutes for it to stand before cutting. We find a great way of serving oven-baked steak is to cut it into very thin slices and serve with fresh horseradish sauce with a little added heavy cream or double cream.

Avocados

A creamy, filling companion

Avocados are a perfect companion to many dishes. They can form part of most dishes that need a little extra bulk. This includes scrambled eggs, prawns with homemade mayonnaise, and herring salad.

Avocados are picked and allowed to ripen at room temperature. You will know that the avocado is ready when it feels slightly soft to the touch. Although it turns from its light green color to black over time, do not be put off with some dark patches that form, as they are safe to eat.

Simply split the avocado long ways and remove the single large stone. When it is ready for consumption, the skin comes off relatively easily.

We recommend that you keep a stock in your kitchen, as they may form a significant part of your diet.

Baked cod cutlets

Light and tasty with delicate flavors
Serves 2

You will need

Baking tray and foil
Takes about 30 minutes in the middle of the oven, at 390ºF,
200ºC or gas mark 6

Ingredients

4 - cod cutlets

Salt and pepper

1 - silver onion

1 - large tomato

4 teaspoons - butter

4 tablespoons - milk

Chopped parsley

Begin

Loosely line the baking tray with foil and leave some extra
at the edge to fold later.
Wash the fish, season with salt and pepper, and place on
the tray.
Peel the onion and slice 4 fairly thin rings, placing 1 on each
cutlet.

Wash the tomato, slice into rings, and place 1 slice on top of each piece of onion.

Put a teaspoon of butter on top of each one and add the milk.

Fold in the foil and close it completely, but leave a space so as not to touch the top of the fish.

Cook in the middle of the oven for about 30 minutes or until soft.

After cooking, the liquid from the foil can be mixed with a little chopped parsley and used as drizzle or decoration before serving.

This is great served with leeks and spinach.

Tip

You can also follow this recipe using plaice; just leave out the onion and tomato.

Stuffed Portobello mushrooms with sausage meat

Filling and super-strong flavors
Serves 2

You will need

Frying pan
Grill tray
Foil

Ingredients

6 - pork sausages, 95 percent meat content
1 tablespoon - ghee or butter
Salt and pepper
4 - large Portobello mushrooms

Begin

Remove skin from the sausages and crumble the meat as best you can. Place the sausage meat in the frying pan with ½ the ghee or butter and salt and pepper to your taste. Leave it to fry off whilst turning occasionally.

Peel the mushrooms, leaving the stalks in place. Put a little of the remaining ghee or butter into each mushroom cap and place on a foiled grill tray.

Fill each mushroom with lots of the meat; really pile it on. Pour the liquid from the frying pan over each mushroom and place under grill.

Grill until mushrooms are soft and the top of the meat goes crispy. Ready to enjoy.

Tip

If you want to add some color, you can decorate with a ring of tomato and grated cheese.

These mushrooms should be eaten hot and make a great breakfast or will go well with any vegetable.

Chicken breasts in butter, garlic, and onion sauce

Butter lovers' delight
Serves 2
Takes about an hour

You will need

Large flat pan

Ingredients

4 tablespoons - ghee or butter

1 - chopped very mild onion

2 - finely chopped garlic cloves

2 - chicken breasts

½ - fresh lemon

1 cup (250 ml) - chicken stock

Begin

Prepare flat pan and heat the ghee or butter.

Chop the onion into thin slices and add to the melted ghee or butter. Cook until they start to become slightly transparent.

Add chopped garlic, stirring continuously until golden brown.

Add chicken breasts until just cooked through.

Squeeze the juice from the lemon into pan and stir around chicken, then add chicken stock.

Bring to the boil, then reduce heat. Stir occasionally so as to avoid sticking.

When the sauce is at the right consistency for your taste, remove from heat and serve with fresh vegetables.

Tip

A little white wine will add to the flavor.

Pickled herring fillets with beetroot and yoghurt

Refreshingly tasty with a creamy texture

You will need

A mixing bowl

Ingredients

8 to 12 - pickled herring fillets

2 - cooked beetroots

18 ounces (500 grams) - Greek full fat yoghurt

Begin

Cut fillets to about 1-inch or 3-centimeter pieces and place in large bowl.

Cut beetroots into mouth-size bites and add to the bowl. (You may want to wear rubber gloves for the beetroot.)

Empty contents of yoghurt into bowl and blend gently.

The color will alter and become a pinky rose.

Serve with celery sticks.

Looks nice presented with some raw beetroot grated on the top just before serving.

Use a lettuce leaf to fill and roll up for a quick and easy hand snack.

Tip

Refrigerating for an hour before serving gives it a cool, fresh taste.

Minced beef in tomato sauce lettuce wrap

Crispy hand rolls with a great meaty taste
Serves 2

You will need

A medium-sized flat pan

Ingredients

1 tablespoon - butter

4 cloves - chopped garlic

18 ounces (500 grams) - minced beef

1 tin - chopped plum tomatoes, (14 ounces or 400 grams)

2 cups (400 ml) - water

1 tablespoon - tomato puree

1 splash - red wine (optional)

1 teaspoon - fresh chopped basil

1 head - iceberg or Chinese leaf lettuce

Begin

Prepare flat pan by heating butter and chopped garlic until golden brown.

Add minced beef slowly and stir until it is cooked through.

Remove the mince from pan, leaving as much of the juice from the mince in the pan as possible.

Add tomatoes and water and bring to boil; add tomato puree, wine and basil and reduce heat.

Stir occasionally until the sauce has reduced to about half its volume, then reintroduce the mince and blend into the sauce.

Wash and separate the lettuce. Use the lettuce leaf as a semi-wrap by spooning the mince onto the lettuce before serving. Roll and munch.

Tip

You can add some grated cheddar cheese or sour cream on top as an extra.

Minced lamb in a creamy curry sauce

Spice lovers' quickie
Serves 4

You will need

A heavy saucepan

Ingredients

1 tablespoon - ghee or butter

6 - finely chopped garlic cloves

18 ounces (500 grams) - minced lamb

3 tablespoons - Madras curry powder

1 tin - chopped plum tomatoes, (14 ounces or 400 grams)

1tablespoon - tomato puree

7 ounces (200 grams) - coconut cream

1tablespoon - fresh chopped coriander

Begin

Prepare flat pan with heated ghee or butter and chopped garlic until golden brown.

Add mince slowly and stir until it is cooked through.

Add curry powder and stir through until the mince is thoroughly covered.

Drop in the tomatoes, add tomato puree and bring to the boil; reduce heat.

Stir occasionally as to avoid sticking.

If necessary, you can add some hot water to create the right texture.

Add coconut cream and, once heated through, add coriander and heat for another few minutes before removing from heat.

Neck of lamb stew

A tasty and filling dish in a rich meat and tomato sauce
Serves 4

You will need

Large, heavy-based saucepan with lid

Ingredients

7 ounces (200 grams) - ghee or butter

4½ pounds (2 kilos) - neck of lamb, including bone

10 ounces (300 grams) - shallots

4 - garlic cloves

2 tins - chopped plum tomatoes (total of 28 ounces or 800 grams)

4 cups (1 liter) - water

3½ ounces (100 grams) - tomato puree

4 - bay leaves

1 teaspoon - cinnamon powder

2 teaspoons - paprika

Begin

Heat half of the ghee or butter in a large saucepan.

Once the pan is hot, start placing the lamb pieces and sear the meat so as it browns.

Remove the meat and set to one side.

Peel shallots and garlic and place in the pot with the remaining ghee or butter.

Stir for about 2 minutes, then add tomatoes.

Mix gently for a minute then reintroduce the lamb and gently stir the mix until lamb is covered.

Add water, tomato puree, bay leaves, cinnamon, and paprika.

Bring to boil and simmer gently for between 1½ and 2 hours, making sure that the stew remains moist.

Add more water if necessary.

If you prefer the stock thicker, once the meat is cooked, remove it from the pan and keep it warm. Increase the heat and allow the stock to gently thicken, then reintroduce the lamb.

Serve on a bed of pureed broccoli with a side dish or fresh french beans.

Tip

Using a pressure cooker reduces the cooking time to 45 minutes and retains more flavor.

Omelet with bacon, cheese, and herbs

A quick meal for breakfast, lunch, or dinner
Serves 1

You will need

Frying pan

Mixing bowl

Ingredients

1 tablespoon - ghee or butter

3 - bacon rashers, sliced into strips

3 - eggs

2 tablespoons - milk

½ tablespoon - fresh parsley

½ tablespoon - fresh chives

4½ ounces (125 grams) - grated cheddar cheese

Begin

Prepare a frying pan by lightly covering the surface with a little of the ghee or butter.

Add bacon and cook until brown and crispy, then remove from pan.

Blend all the eggs, milk, parsley and chives gently in a bowl.

Heat the remaining ghee or butter in a flat pan.

Pour egg mixture into pan and cook until the top is almost set and the underside starts to brown.

Gently flip it over to cook the other side. Add grated cheese.

Then tip bacon mix on half of the surface and fold over.

Cook until omelet is brown on both sides.

Garnish with salad or avocado and serve.

Perfect scrambled eggs

Smooth and creamy

You will need

A mixing bowl

A shallow pan

Ingredients

3½ ounces (100 grams) - butter

3 - fresh eggs per person

Salt and pepper to taste

Begin

Heat pan and add butter.

Blend eggs until yolk is fully mixed.

Add salt and pepper.

Gently pour in blended eggs.

Keep gently mixing whilst cooking until the texture is creamy and smooth.

Ensure that the mix is just cooked through to retain the buttery taste.

Tip

Serve with ripe avocado and bacon or sausages.

Prawn and salmon lettuce rolls

A mouthwatering extravaganza of seafood and mayonnaise

You will need

Saucepan for hot water

A bowl for cold water

Clean, flat surface

Make 1 hour before serving

Serves 2

Serve cold

Ingredients

1 large - iceberg or cos lettuce

4 - celery sticks

1 tablespoon - capers

9 ounces (250 grams) - fresh salmon (can be replaced by crab meat)

9 ounces (250 grams) - cooked fresh prawns—medium sized

3½ ounces - (100 grams) mayonnaise

Pinch - dill weed

Ground fresh pepper and salt if necessary

Begin

Prepare a saucepan of hot water and a bowl of cold water.
Separate and wash lettuce leaves. Best to use the larger leaves and leave the small ones for garnish.
Place the larger leaves in hot water and leave until stem softens, 1 to 2 minutes.
Remove and place in bowl of cold water.
Wash celery and remove stringy bits; cut into small pieces.
Chop capers into small pieces.
Prepare salmon by steaming or boiling until cooked through.
Chop prawns into small pieces.
Once salmon is cooled, crumble it and mix with prawns and celery.
Add mayonnaise, dill weed, capers, and pepper and salt into mix, then blend gently with hands.
Separate the lettuce leaves and individually place on a flat surface.
Take a spoonful of the prawn and salmon mix and place on a lettuce leaf so that it can be rolled evenly.
Fold edges into roll where possible.
Once completed, place the filled rolls into container and refrigerate for at least 1 hour.
Serve with a twist of lemon and salad garnish.

Super-duper brussels sprouts

Flavorsome with strong, earthy taste.
Full of flavor
Serves 2

You will need

Saucepan
Takes about 30 minutes

Ingredients

10 ounces (300 grams) - brussels sprouts

2 tablespoons - ghee or butter

1 - clove garlic

Salt and pepper

Begin

Fill the saucepan with enough water to cover the sprouts and add a small ½ teaspoon of salt.
Put the water on to boil and start to prepare the sprouts by washing and cutting them in half.
When the water boils, add the sprouts, bring back to the boil, turn down heat, and simmer for 10 minutes.
After 10 minutes, drain sprouts and remove from pan; add ghee or butter and garlic to warm empty pan, and put pan back on heat.

Add sprouts, salt, and pepper, and cook over a high heat; keep turning till slightly brown. They're ready.

If you like pepper, you can add quite a lot to this dish. It works well.

Tip

You can add a teaspoon of quality fermented soy sauce at the frying-off stage to give it a unique flavor.

Also

It is also nice to cook cabbage in this style. Chop the cabbage quite thick, though.

Cauliflower with cheese

Gets the taste buds going
Serves 2

You will need

Large saucepan
Ovenproof dish
Cheese grater

Ingredients

¼ teaspoon - salt
18 ounces (500 grams) - cauliflower florets
7 ounces (200 grams) - cheddar or similar strong cheese
Pepper

Begin

Put a large pan of water on to boil, adding ¼ teaspoon of salt.
Remove outer leaves and stalk of cauliflower and discard.
Wash florets and drop them into the boiling, salty water.
Reduce heat and let it simmer for 15 minutes or until softened.
When the cauliflower is cooked, drain and place florets into ovenproof dish.
Grate the cheese all over the cauliflower, sprinkle on some pepper, and place it under the grill.
Cook until cheese bubbles and goes brown.

Tip

You can be as wild as you like with the cheese; add as much as you like and even explore with different types of cheeses.

Spinach, yoghurt, cucumber, and garlic filler

A zing with freshness

You will need

A large mixing bowl

Ingredients

9 ounces (250 grams) - spinach leaves

9 ounces (250 grams) – full-fat plain yoghurt

1 clove - garlic, cleaned and crushed

½ - cucumber, peeled and chopped

Fresh pepper to taste

Begin

Wash and tear spinach into yoghurt with garlic, cucumber, and pepper.
Gently blend until the yogurt has fully covered the spinach.

Tip

Use to fill avocados or as a side dish.

Yoghurt and heavy cream or double cream dessert

Ideal for dessert, breakfast, or as a snack

Blend a mix of approximately 10 ounces (300 milliliters) of full-fat yoghurt with 10 ounces (300 milliliters) of heavy or double cream.

Prepare your favorite ripe fruit from the approved list and mix.

Seasonal fruit is recommended, particularly soft fruits that are local to your area.

Three Tasty Treat Recipes

Whilst your goal is to lose weight, it is important to minimize starchy ingredients. An occasional dish that includes potatoes or white rice is acceptable for some dieters, so long as you control the portion size. Here are three such recipes.

Liver, bacon, and kidneys

Mighty, meaty, and very tasty
Serves 2

You will need

Large plate
Flat pan
Ovenproof dish with lid

Takes about an hour at 390ºF, 200ºC or gas mark 6, in the middle of the oven

Ingredients

5 tablespoons - potato flour

Salt and pepper

4 - lambs' kidneys

18 ounces (500 grams) - lambs liver

1 teaspoon - ghee or butter

1 - onion

6 rashers - smoked streaky bacon

1 tin - chopped tomatoes (14 ounces or 400 grams)

Begin

Spread the flour around the plate and sprinkle with salt and pepper.

Wash the kidneys and the liver.

Cut the kidneys in half and remove white gristle.

Roll the kidneys and liver in the flour, salt, and pepper until completely covered.

Heat the ghee or butter in the pan and gently sear the kidneys and liver.

Finely chop the onion and sprinkle over the base of the oven dish. Add the cooked meat, rashers of bacon, and tin of tomatoes.

The liquid needs to cover the meat, so add a little water if required.

Put the lid on and place in the middle of the oven for about an hour.

Jacket potatoes royal

Ultimate jackets with a crispy exterior and a fluffy centre

You will need

2 long skewers
Takes about 2 hours in the middle of the oven at 430ºF,
220ºC or gas mark 7

Ingredients

4 large - baking potatoes
Goose fat
Salt

Begin

Wash the potatoes and put 2 on each skewer.
Smother with goose fat and salt.
Place in middle of oven for 2 hours.

Tip

Goes with most main courses, or fill with your favorite
topping. How about some smoked salmon with cream
cheese, or sour cream and chives or bacon? You can always
add tuna with celery. The choices are endless.

Extra Tip

When potatoes are cold, you can slice and fry in ghee or
butter. They can last up to three days in the refrigerator
once baked.

Creamy cabbage
Luxury vegetable to diet for
Serves 2

You will need

2 large saucepans

Ingredients

¼ teaspoon - salt

7 ounces (200 grams) - cabbage

2 tablespoons - ghee or butter

Pepper

2 large - potatoes

7 ounces (200 milliliters) – heavy or double cream

Begin

Fill a large saucepan with cold water. Add ¼ teaspoon of salt and place on hob to boil.

Discard the outer leaves and stalk of the cabbage and finely chop remainder.

When water boils, drop in the chopped cabbage and let it cook for 10 minutes or until soft.

When the cabbage is cooked, drain off the water and add 1 tablespoon of ghee or butter to the empty saucepan.

Tip the drained cabbage into the ghee and stir well, adding plenty of pepper. Put to one side.

Peel and cut potatoes into 8 pieces.

Place potatoes in saucepan of cold water, enough to cover the potatoes; add ¼ teaspoon salt and bring to the boil.

Once boiling, let them cook for 15 minutes or until soft enough to mash.

When the potatoes are cooked, drain off the water, add 1 tablespoon of ghee or butter to the empty saucepan, and mash the potatoes until they are broken down and well blended with the ghee.

Blend cabbage and potatoes together and slowly add the cream.

It is now ready to serve with your chosen dish.

Tip

If you have any left over, it fries up really well in ghee or butter. Fry until brown and crispy, turning occasionally. You can have it with your breakfast eggs and bacon.

Glossary

Absurd magical beliefs—the ability to imagine logical outcomes based on an illogical premise. (If I avoid the cracks on the pavement, Mummy will not shout at me for not doing my homework.)

Addiction—a psychological or physiological dependence to a substance or state of being.

Adiponectin—a hormone released by fat cells that controls the metabolism of fats and glucose. In addition, adiponectin has a role in the body's response to insulin release and acts as an anti-inflammatory on the cells of blood vessels.

Adipose tissue—body fat.

Adrenaline (also known as epinephrine)—produced by the adrenal glands and released in response to various stresses. It is both a hormone and a neurotransmitter, and its effects include contraction of blood vessels, increase in heart rate, and dilation of air passages. Its effects are noticeable in the "fight or flight response."

Affirmation—a declaration of truth. Often used in self-help as a statement to positively program the subconscious mind.

Agricultural Revolution—also known as the First Agricultural Revolution or the Neolithic Revolution.

Happened around ten thousand years ago and represents a major move away from the fat- and protein-based hunter-gatherer diet to a diet that began to include more cereal grains and domesticated crops.

Alkylresorcinols—a type of lipid (fat) found in whole wheat and whole rye.

Amino acids—the precursor building blocks of proteins.

Amygdala—the part of the brain responsible for processing (and recalling) emotional reactions.

Anchors—based on Pavlovian research, anchors are stimuli that trigger a response. For example, if someone holds his or her hand out as a handshake, we are anchored to responding likewise.

Antinutrients—compounds, found in certain foods, which interfere with the absorption of beneficial nutrients.

Antioxidants—naturally occurring substances in foods that *may* help protect our cells from damage caused by free radicals (molecules produced by the body during digestion of foods and exposure to environmental stresses).

Artificial sweeteners—man-made, chemical sweeteners that include saccharin, aspartame, acesulfame-K, and sucralose.

Atherosclerosis—a condition in which plaque builds up in the walls of the arteries. This plaque hardens, causing a narrowing of the arteries with the effect of limiting the flow of blood through them.

Autoimmune disorders—diseases where the body's immune system attacks its own cells. Crohns Disease, diabetes mellitus type 1 and Hashimoto's thyroiditis are examples of autoimmune disorders.

Beliefs—information either internally or externally generated that the mind accepts as being true.

Blood pressure—the pressure of the blood circulating through the blood vessels. A typical reading is 120/80—the first number represents the pressure of the blood moving away from the heart, and the second number, the pressure of the blood as it returns to the heart.

Blood sugar—glucose, the primary energy source for the cells of the body.

Blood sugar levels—the amount of glucose present in the blood.

Body fat—also known as adipose tissue, this is the body's stored fat energy that also serves as insulation and protective padding. It consists of subcutaneous fat (the layer beneath the skin), visceral fat (around the internal organs), and breast tissue.

Buy-in loop—when an individual or corporation has established a relationship that fosters a sense of obligation to the purchase of a product or service.

Caffeine—an alkaloid traditionally present in drinks like tea and coffee; has a stimulant effect.

Calorie restriction—a form of diet where calories are usually counted and food intake deliberately controlled to ensure only a certain target number of calories is consumed.

Calories—in nutrition, this refers to the kilocalorie (kcal), a unit of measurement of the energy value of foods.

Carbohydrates—a macronutrient food group that includes simple sugars and more complex starches.

Carbs—common abbreviation for the term "carbohydrates." See "carbohydrates."

Cardiovascular—relating to the human cardiovascular system. The heart pumps blood through the blood vessels, the blood is oxygenated via the lungs, and this oxygenated blood is used throughout the body.

Cardiovascular disease—also known as heart disease, most commonly used to refer to atherosclerosis (see separate entry).

Casein—a type of protein found in milk and cheese.

Cereals—grasses that have been cultivated for their seed head, particularly since the First Agricultural Revolution. The seed head is then used in a multitude of foods in either its whole grain form or after being refined. Common cereals include corn/maize, rice, wheat, barley, oats, and rye.

Cerebral artery disease—disease affecting an artery within the brain or that supplies the brain. Includes atherosclerosis and defects or weaknesses in a blood vessel of the brain. Also known as cerebrovascular disease.

Cholesterol—a naturally occurring steroid that carries out many vital functions. Most cholesterol is made within the body in the liver and other tissues; the rest is derived from dietary intake. Circulates in the blood as lipoproteins— HDL, high-density lipoproteins; LDL, low-density lipoproteins; and VLDL, very low-density lipoproteins.

Cholesterol levels—measurement of the amount of total blood cholesterol, including high-density lipoproteins, low-density lipoproteins, and very low-density lipoproteins.

Common sense—seen as an ability that is acquired through childhood learning and development, common sense allows for the practical solution to a situation.

Compulsion—an inability to avoid an action or behavior in spite of the outcome.

Coronary artery disease (CAD)—hardening and narrowing of the arteries that supply blood to the heart.

Deletion—the unconscious process whereby one excludes a portion of an experience or a remembered thought.

Diabetes—*diabetes mellitus*. A group of diseases related to the glucose metabolism, including type 1 diabetes, type 2 diabetes, and gestational diabetes. A person with diabetes has high blood sugar levels due to either the body not producing enough insulin or because the cells have become resistant to the insulin that is produced.

Diet pill—any pill that claims to aid weight loss, often based on a form of stimulant.

Disaccharides—a carbohydrate/sugar consisting of two monosaccharides joined together. Includes sucrose (table sugar) and lactose (milk sugar).

Distortion—the unconscious process whereby a current or remembered event is changed to fit one's existing model of the world.

Docosahexaenoic acid (DHA)—an omega-3 fatty acid present in fish oils, eggs, and meat from cattle reared on grass.

Drivers—the underlying force that motivates action.

Ectomorph—one of the three somatotypes. An ectomorphic body shape is typically long and lean with naturally low body fat levels.

Eicosapentaenoic acid (EPA) — an omega-3 fatty acid present in oily fish, fish oils, and human breast milk.

Endomorph — one of the three somatotypes. An endomorphic body shape is typically rounded with higher body fat levels.

Epigenetics — the study of how gene expression changes without alteration to the underlying genetic code. Stress, diet, and other environmental factors affect the epigenome (a set of biochemical modifications on the genome which modify the genetic instructions), switching genes on or off, or increasing or decreasing their influence.

Epinephrine — see "Adrenaline."

Essential amino acids — amino acids that cannot be synthesized by the human body and must be provided in the diet.

Exercise — physical activity carried out with the purpose of improving or optimizing the functioning and/or appearance of the body.

Fast-fattening foods — sugars, refined carbohydrates, rapidly digested carbohydrates, and foods containing the aforementioned.

Fasting — a period of time where consumption of energy (food and calorific drinks) is deliberately avoided.

Fat burning—switching the body into a state where more body fat is being utilized for energy than is being stored.

Fat-free—a term used for processed foods and drinks where naturally occurring fats have been removed from the end product.

Fatty acids—types of molecule in fats, oils, and cell membranes that are a component of glycolipids and phosopholipids. Includes cis and trans unsaturated fatty acids, saturated fatty acids and essential fatty acids.

Fiber—indigestible carbohydrates which may be soluble (e.g., pectin in fruit) or insoluble (e.g., cellulose in plants). Sources of dietary fiber include fruit, vegetables, and nuts.

Food diary—a journal for keeping track of daily food and drink intake.

Fructose—a simple monosaccharide sugar that naturally occurs in fruit, honey, and some root vegetables.

Generalization—the unconscious process whereby a single event or a few events are taken to indicate how all similar events will result.

Ghee—a clarified butter that is nearly pure fat.

GI tract—short for gastrointestinal tract, the long tube and connected organs that start at the mouth and end at the anus. This includes the mouth, esophagus, stomach, small intestine, large intestine/colon, and anus.

Glucose—blood sugar.

Glucose syrup—a sweetener derived from starch.

Gluten—a protein composite derived mainly from wheat, barley, and rye.

Glycemic control—management of glucose levels in the blood.

Glycerol—a compound that is the "backbone" to all triglycerides.

Glycogen—a quickly mobilized form of energy converted from glucose and stored in the body as a reserve.

Grain fed—animals that have been fed grain as opposed to grass; very common as a modern farming practice.

Grain oil—oil derived from grain crops like corn.

Grains—see "Cereals."

Grass fed—animals that have been fed a natural diet of grass, producing the healthiest meat.

Growth hormone—a hormone produced by the anterior pituitary gland. Its effects include strengthening of the bones, increasing of muscle mass, promoting the breakdown of fats, and stimulating the immune system, among many other functions.

Habits—patterns of repeated behavior usually only recognized when a sequence has been disrupted. For example, when we move the cupboards around, it takes a few days to create new patterns, which then become habits.

Heart disease—a term that encompasses the different diseases of the heart. These include coronary heart disease, cardiomyopathy, cardiovascular disease, ischemic heart disease, heart failure, hypertensive heart disease, inflammatory heart disease, and valvular heart disease.

High-density lipoprotein (HDL)—the lipoprotein sometimes referred to as "good cholesterol." Its role is to carry cholesterol, triglycerides, and lipids to the liver via blood. HDL contains a higher proportion of protein and has a smaller particle size compared to other lipoproteins.

High fat diet—a diet where the majority of calories/energy is derived from fat. In addition, high fat diets usually have a moderate protein intake and a minimal carbohydrate intake.

High fructose corn syrup (also called glucose-fructose syrup)—a highly refined sweetener found in many processed foods and drinks.

High intensity strength training—a form of exercise that improves the function of the musculature, the cardiovascular system, and all the body's supporting systems. Also raises the metabolic rate, aiding in weight loss and appearance goals.

Hormone sensitive lipase—the main enzyme responsible for the mobilization of fatty acids from adipose (fat) tissue.

Hormones—the powerful chemical messengers of the body. Hormones are made in the endocrine glands and travel through the bloodstream to organs and tissues, where they influence many processes throughout the body, including metabolism, growth, mood, and sexual function.

Hunter-Gatherer—a society or member of a society whose primary methods of attaining food are hunting animals and foraging plants from the wild.

Hydrogenated fat—a fat that has undergone the hydrogenation process, suiting food producers because of the resulting extended shelf and/or fry life of the fat. Found in many processed food products. Unhealthy for the human metabolism.

Insulin—a major nutrient storage hormone, the main role of insulin being to process glucose out of the blood.

Insulin sensitivity—normal functioning of the body in response to the release of insulin. Conversely, when a person becomes insulin resistant, greater amounts of insulin are released by the pancreas in an attempt to process glucose; this leads to health issues.

Interesterified fat—a form of hydrogenated fat.

Intermittent fasting—periods of time where a person deliberately avoids caloric intake to boost weight loss results.

Internal starvation—a negative metabolic effect where the body by default shuttles most of its incoming food energy straight to fat storage.

IU (International Unit)—a measurement of the biological activity of a substance, e.g., 1,000 IU of vitamin D3.

Kaka—a term to denote any form of junk food/fluid, or "miracle" weight loss product.

Ketogenic—refers to a diet that stimulates the production of ketones.

Ketones—chemicals produced in the body when fat is broken down to provide energy.

Ketosis—the state where ketones are being produced by the body.

Lactose—a form of naturally occurring sugar found primarily in milk. Some people are intolerant to lactose.

Lauric acid—a saturated fatty acid found in human breast milk and coconut oil that aids the immune system.

Lectins—carbohydrate-binding proteins primarily found in beans and cereal grains that may cause gastrointestinal distress, allergic reactions, and nutritional deficiencies. They have also been indicated as a possible cause of obesity.

Leptin—a hormone that plays a major part in regulating energy intake and expenditure, it affects both metabolism and appetite.

Lipids—various molecules that include fats/triglycerides, fatty acids, and cholesterol.

Lipolysis—the breakdown of lipids, including stored body fat being used for energy.

Low calorie diet—see "Calorie restriction."

Low-density lipoprotein (LDL)—one of the types of lipoproteins whose role is to carry water-insoluble lipids in the bloodstream.

Low fat—a term used for processed foods and drinks where naturally occurring fats have been largely removed from the end product.

Low fat diet—a form of diet in which a key focus is keeping fat intake minimal.

Macronutrients—the three major energy sources in the human diet: fats, proteins and carbohydrates.

Maltodextrin—a highly processed food additive sweetener, found in many processed foods and drinks.

Mesomorph—one of the three somatotypes. A mesomorphic body shape is typically muscular in appearance, with wide shoulders and a relatively low amount of body fat.

Metabolic rate—the rate at which the body burns calories for energy.

Metabolic syndrome—a collection of interrelated diseases, conditions, and health issues caused primarily by the modern diet. Some individuals may be more genetically predisposed to developing metabolic syndrome than others.

Modeling—a key neurolinguistic process whereby one can elicit the essence of the ideas or thoughts someone has to achieve a goal. This can then be taught to others.

Monosaccharides—the simplest form of sugars; includes glucose, galactose, and fructose.

Norepinephrine—one of the "fight or flight" hormones that are released by the adrenal glands.

Ob gene—the gene responsible for encoding the hormone leptin.

Obesity—accumulation of excess body fat to the point where there may be a development of negative effects on the health of the individual.

Obsessive behaviors—an inability to detach from an action or idea in the belief that something disastrous would occur.

Omega-3—a group of unsaturated fatty acids which most people in the modern Western world do not consume enough of.

Omega-6—a group of unsaturated fatty acids that most people in the modern Western world consume too much of.

Osteoarthritis—a degenerative joint disease.

Outcome—the result of an action.

Paleolithic—the era of human prehistory denoted by the first known use of stone tools, from some 2.6 million years ago until the commencement of agriculture about twelve thousand years ago. During this time period humans lived primarily as hunter-gatherers.

Pasteurized—a food (most commonly milk) that has been heated to a specific temperature for a certain length of time, destroying its bacteria.

Pastured—animals that have been allowed to graze/feed on a diet of grass (as opposed to grain fed).

Pesticide—a substance or combination of substances typically applied to crops to destroy pests or prevent damage caused by pests. Widely used in modern agriculture.

Phytates—phosphorus stored in plant tissues that, when consumed by humans, binds to important minerals like magnesium, calcium, zinc, and iron, rendering them nonabsorbable by the intestines, acting in these cases as an antinutrient.

Plant oils—oils derived from grains, seeds, nuts, and some fruits.

Polysaccharides—complex sugars also known as starches.

Polyunsaturated fats—the primary polyunsaturated fats are omega-3 and omega-6, which are essential fatty acids that must be derived from the diet, as the body cannot manufacture them.

Protease inhibitors—molecules that stop enzymes from degrading proteins.

Protein—one of the three macronutrients in our diet, protein is considered a building block of life, as it is essential for cell growth and tissue repair. Proteins are made up of amino acids.

Rapidly digested carbohydrates—primarily sugars found in whole foods and added to processed foods. They are digested and absorbed very quickly.

Raw honey—pure, unpasteurized, unheated, and unprocessed honey has health benefits that typical processed honey doesn't.

Reduced-fat—a term used for processed foods and drinks where naturally occurring fats have been somewhat removed from the end product.

Refined carbohydrates—carbohydrates that have been processed; includes sugars, grain flours, and many products that contain these ingredients. One of the major causes of weight gain.

Resistance exercise—strength training.

Resting energy expenditure—the amount of energy (usually measured in calories) that a person requires to drive all his or her physiological processes whilst he or she is inactive/at rest.

Rheumatoid arthritis—an autoimmune disease and systemic inflammatory disorder that primarily affects synovial joints (but can affect other tissues and organs too).

Rituals—symbolic expressions.

Saturated fat—a type of fat made up of triglycerides, which just contain saturated fatty acid radicals. Found primarily in animal fats and dairy products.

Serum triglyceride levels—the amount of triglycerides in the blood.

Smoke point—the temperature at which a cooking oil or fat breaks down to glycerol and free fatty acids. Avoid heating a fat or oil to its smoke point, as it becomes far less healthy to consume.

Somatotypes—the general structure or build of an individual. There are three main somatotypes or body shapes: ectomorph, endomorph, and mesomorph.

Starch—a carbohydrate most notably found in grains and root vegetables.

Stress—the psychological and physiological effects experienced when an individual's resources are challenged.

Sucrose—common table sugar.

Sugars—carbohydrates whose categories include monosaccharides, disaccharides, and polysaccharides.

Sweeteners—natural or artificial food additives that add a sweet flavor.

Syndrome X—see "Metabolic syndrome."

Systemic inflammation—a condition where immune cells release pro- inflammatories and the immune system is chronically activated.

T cell—a type of white blood cell that plays a major role in cell-based immune response.

Thyroid—an endocrine gland located in the neck that produces thyroid hormones responsible for regulating the metabolism.

Trans fat—a type of fat notably found in oils and fats that have been hydrogenated.

Triacylglycerol—the scientific name for triglycerides.

Triggers—stimuli that provoke predetermined responses.

Triglyceride metabolism—see "Lipolysis."

Triglycerides—a form of fat made up of three molecules of fatty acid and a molecule of glycerol. The main kind of fat/lipid stored in the human body as well as animal and vegetable cells.

Type 1 diabetes—type of diabetes where the body fails to produce enough insulin.

Type 2 diabetes—type of diabetes where cells become resistant to the effects of released insulin.

Unsaturated fat—a type of fat that is usually liquid at room temperature, most commonly associated with vegetable oils.

Values—the benefits we are driven towards.

Vegetable oil—oil derived from a plant source.

Visceral fat—the fat that surrounds the internal organs.

Vitamin A—a fat-soluble vitamin that is beneficial for the immune system, the skin, and vision.

Vitamin D—a fat-soluble vitamin that the body can produce naturally with exposure to sufficiently intense sunlight. A very important steroid vitamin that can boost immunity, amongst many other important effects.

Vitamin K2—a fat-soluble vitamin that helps produce blood clotting factors and is involved in strengthening the capillaries and bones.

Water retention—excess accumulation of water in the body.

Yo-yo dieting—a continual cycle of weight loss followed by weight gain.

References

Chapter 1

1. D. E. Pankevich et al., "Caloric restriction experience reprograms stress and orexigenic pathways and promotes binge eating," *J Neurosci*, 2010, 30(48): p. 16399-407.

2. A. Keys, J. Brozek, A. Henschel, et al., *The Biology of Human Starvation* (Minneapolis, MN: University of Minnesota Press, 1950.

Chapter 3

1. Center for Science in the Public Interest, "America: Drowning in Sugar," http://www.cspinet.org/new/sugar.html.

 2. J. H. O'keefe, Jr., and L. Cordain, "Cardiovascular disease resulting from a diet and lifestyle at odds with our paleolithic genome: how to become a 21st-century hunter-gatherer," *Mayo clin proc* 2004 jan;79(1):101-8.; http://www.thepaleodiet.com/index.shtml, retrieved September 15, 2010.

3. Food Inc., 2009.

4. R. H. Eckel et al., "The metabolic syndrome," *Lancet*, 2010, 375: p. 181-3.; X. Lu et al., "Varients in the insulin-degrading enzyme gene are associated with metabolic syndrome in Chinese elders," *Metabolism: clinical and experimental*, 2009, 58:

p. 1465-9.; A. Misra et al., "Novel phenotypic markers and screening score for the metabolic syndrome in adult Asian Indians," *Diabetes research and clinical practice*, 2008, 79: p. E 1-5.; R. L. Pollex et al., "Metabolic syndrome in aboriginal Canadians: prevalence and genetic associations," *Atherosclerosis*, 2006, 184(1): p. 121-9.; G. M. Reaven, "Why Syndrome X? From Harold Himsworth to the insulin resistance syndrome," *Cell metabolism*, 2005, 1: p. 9-14.; M. P. Reilly and D. J. Rader, "The metabolic syndrome: more than the sum of its parts?" *Circulation*, 2003, 108: p. 1546-51.; M. E. Trujillo and P. E. Scherer, "Adiponectin—journey from an adipocyte secretory protein to biomarker of the metabolic syndrome," *Journal of Internal Medicine*, 2005, 257: p. 167-75.

5. W. A. Price, *Nutrition and Physical Degeneration*, 8th ed., 2008, Price-Pottenger Nutrition Foundation. S. Lindeberg et al., "Biological and Clinical Potential of a Palaeolithic Diet," *Journal of Nutritional and Environmental Medicine*, September 2003, 13(3), 149-160.; Cordain Loren, S. Boyd Eaton, Anthony Sebastian, Neil Mann, Staffan Lindeberg, Bruce A. Watkins, James H. O'Keefe, and Janette Brand Miller, "Origins and evolution of the western diet: Health implications for the 21st century," *Am J Clin Nutr* 2005;81:341-54.

6. Jeff S. Volek and Richard D Feinman, "Carbohydrate restriction improves the features of Metabolic Syndrome. Metabolic Syndrome may be defined by the response to carbohydrate restriction," *USA Nutrition & Metabolism*

2005, 2:31doi:10.1186/1743-7075-2-31, http://www.nutritionandmetabolism.com/content/2/1/31.

7. R. Spangler, K. M. Wittkowski, N. L. Goddard, N. M. Avena, B. G. Hoebel, and S. F. Leibowitz, "Opiate-like effects of sugar on gene expression in reward areas of the rat brain," Brain Res Mol Brain Res. 2004 May 19;124(2):134-42.; *Neurosci Biobehav Rev*, 2008; 32(1): 20–39. Published online May 18, 2007, doi: 10.1016/j.neubiorev.2007.04.019.; Nicole M. Avena, Pedro Rada, and Bartley G. Hoebel, "Evidence for sugar addiction: Behavioral and neurochemical effects of intermittent, excessive sugar intake."

8. "Body by Science," Especially for Women, http://www.bodybyscience.net/home.html/?page_id=301.

9. "Body by Science," Especially for Women, http://www.bodybyscience.net/home.html/?page_id=301.

10. L. Cordain, "Cereal grains: humanity's double edged sword," *World Rev Nutr Diet* 1999; 84:19-73.

11.Ibid.

12. T. Stockdale, "A discussion of the relationship between selenium, thyroxine, and indigestion," *Nutr Health*, 1998;12(2):131-4.

13. Figures from Food and Agriculture Organization of the United Nations, 2008 figures, http://faostat.fao.org.

14.
http://en.wikipedia.org/wiki/Agricultural_subsidy#Impact_
on_nutrition.

15. Kimber L. Stanhope, Jean Marc Schwarz, Nancy L.
Keim, Steven C. Griffen, Andrew A. Bremer, James L.
Graham, Bonnie Hatcher, et al., "Consuming fructose-
sweetened, not glucose-sweetened, beverages increases
visceral adiposity and lipids and decreases insulin
sensitivity in overweight/obese humans," *J. Clin.
Invest*, 2009; 119(5):1322.

16. Lois Rogers, "Child diabetes blamed on food
sweetener," The *Sunday Times*, December 13, 2009.

17. Sharon S. Elliott, Nancy L. Keim, Judith S. Stern, Karen
Teff, and Peter J Havel, "Fructose, weight gain, and the
insulin resistance syndrome," *Am J Clin Nutr* 79 (4): 537–
43.PMID 15051594, April 2004.

18. Chi-Tang Ho et al., *ScienceDaily*, August 23, 2007,
http://www.sciencedaily.com/releases/2007/08/07082309481
9.htm.

19. Renee Dufault, Blaise LeBlanc, Roseanne Schnoll, et
al. (2009), "Mercury from chlor-alkali plants: measured
concentrations in food product sugar," *Environmental
Health* 8: 2.doi:10.1186/1476-069X-8-
2. PMID 19171026. PMC 2637263.

20. R. A. Forshee, M. L. Storey, D. B. Allison, W. H. Glinsmann, G. L. Hein, D. R. Lineback, S. A. Miller, T. A. Nicklas, et al. (2007), "A critical examination of the evidence relating high fructose corn syrup and weight gain."; P. Monsivais et al. (2007), "Sugars and satiety: does the type of sweetener make a difference?" *American Journal of Clinical Nutrition* 86 (1): 116–123.

21. Susan E. Swithers and Terry L. Davidson, "A Role for Sweet Taste: Calorie Predictive Relations in Energy Regulation by Rats," *Purdue University Behavioral Neuroscience* 2008, Vol. 122, No. 1, 161–173.

22. http://www.uthscsa.edu/hscnews/singleformat2.asp?newID =1539, retrieved October 8, 2010.

23. T. Just, H. W. Pau, U. Engel, T. Hummel, "Cephalic phase insulin release in healthy humans after taste stimulation?" *Appetite*, 2008, Nov;51(3):622-7. E-pub May 10, 2008.

24. "All About Genetically Modified Foods," http://kroger.staywellsolutionsonline.com/Library/News/1, 2870, retrieved September 20, 2010.

Chapter 4

1. U. Ravnskov, "The questionable role of saturated and polyunsaturated fatty acids in cardiovascular disease," *Clin Epidemiol* 1998 Jun;51(6):443-60.; A. Mente, L. de Koning, H. S.

Shannon, and S. S. Anand, "A systematic review of the evidence supporting a causal link between dietary factors and coronary heart disease," *Arch Intern Med* 2009 Apr 13;169(7):659-69.; Paul Oglesby, MD, Mark H. Lepper, MD, William H. Phelan, MD, G. Wesley Dupertuis, PhD, Anne Macmillan, BSc, Harlley Mckean, PhD, Heebok Park, MS, "A Longitudinal Study of Coronary Heart Disease," *Circulation* 1963;28:20.; J. N. Morris, J. W. Marr, and D. G. Clayton, "Diet and heart: a postscript," *Br Med J,* 1977 November 19; 2(6098): 1307–1314.

2. The Weston A. Price Foundation, "Know Your Fats Introduction," 2009, http://www.westonaprice.org/know-your-fats/561-know-your-fats-introduction.html, retrieved September 20, 2010.

3. E. M. Cranton, MD, and J. P. Frackelton, MD, *Journal of Holistic Medicine,* Spring/Summer 1984, Nutrition Week, March 22, 1991 21:12:2-3.

4. C. V. Felton, D. Crook, M. J. Davies, and M. F. Oliver, "Dietary polyunsaturated fatty acids and composition of human aortic plaques," Volume 344, Issue 8931, October 29, 1994, pages 1195-1196.

5. http://www.westonaprice.org/know-your-fats/526-skinny-on-fats.html, 2000.

6. Statins and the Cholesterol Hypothesis – Part I Kurt G Harris MD http://www.paleonu.com/panu-

weblog/2010/7/21/statins-and-the-cholesterol-hypothesis-part-i.html retrieved March 2nd 2011

7. http://www.framinghamheartstudy.org/about/history.html, retrieved September 20, 2010.

8. Tavia Gordon, William P. Castelli, Marthana C. Hjortland, William B. Kannel, and Thomas R. Dawber, "High density lipoprotein as a protective factor against coronary heart disease: The Framingham study," *The American Journal of Medicine*, May 1977, Vol. 62, Issue 5, Pages 707-714.

9. "Principles of Healthy Diets," http://www.westonaprice.org/abcs-of-nutrition/475-principles-of-healthy-diets.html, retrieved September 20, 2010.

10. H. Edward Garrett, MD, Evan C. Horning, PhD, Billy G. Creech, PhD, Michael De Bakey, MD, "Serum Cholesterol Values in Patients Treated Surgically for Atherosclerosis," *JAMA*, 1964;189(9):655-659.

11. A. W. Weverling-Rijnsburger, G. J. Blauw, A. M. Lagaay, D. L. Knook, A. E. Meinders, and R. G. Westendorp, "Total cholesterol and risk of mortality in the oldest old," *Lancet*, 1997 Oct 18;350(9085):1119-23.

12. Harlan M. Krumholz, MD, Teresa E. Seeman, PhD, Susan S. Merrill, PhD, Carlos F. Mendes de Leon, PhD, Viola Vaccarino, MD, David I. Silverman, MD, Reiko Tsukahara, MD, Adrian

M. Ostfeld, MD, and Lisa F. Berkman, PhD, "Lack of Association Between Cholesterol and Coronary Heart Disease Mortality and Morbidity and All-Cause Mortality in Persons Older Than 70 Years," *JAMA*, 1994;272(17):1335-1340. doi:10.1001/jama.1994.03520170045034.

13. D. Mozaffarian, M. B. Katan, A. Ascherio, M. J. Stampfer, W. C. Willett (2006), "Trans fatty acids and cardiovascular disease," *N Engl J Med*, 354 (15): 1601–13.

14. V. A. Chajès, C. M. Thiébaut, M. Rotival, E. Gauthier, V. Maillard, M. C. Boutron-Ruault, V. Joulin, G. M. Lenoir, F. Clavel-Chapelon (2008), "Serum trans-monounsaturated fatty acids are associated with an increased risk of breast cancer in the E3N-EPIC Study," *Am J Epidemiol* 167 (11): 1312.

15. K. Kavanagh, K. L. Jones, J. Sawyer, K. Kelley, J. J. Carr, J. D. Wagner, L. L. Rudel (July 15, 2007), "Trans fat diet induces abdominal obesity and changes in insulin sensitivity in monkeys," *Obesity* (Silver Spring), 15 (7): 1675–84.

16. M. Mahfouz, (1981), "Effect of dietary trans fatty acids on the delta 5, delta 6 and delta 9 desaturases of rat liver microsomes in vivo." *Acta biologica et medica germanica* 40 (12): 1699–1705.

17. K. Sundram, T. Karupaiah, and K. Hayes (2007), "Stearic acid-rich interesterified fat and trans-rich

fat raise the LDL/HDL ratio and plasma glucose relative to palm olein in humans," *Nutr Metab* 4: 3.

18. I. E. Liener (1994), "Implications of antinutritional components in soybean foods," *Crit Rev Food Sci Nutr*, vol. 34, pp. 31-67.; Y. P. Gupta (1987), "Antinutritional and toxic factors in food legumes: a review," *Plant Foods for Human Nutrition*, vol. 37, pp. 201-228.; N. D. Noah et al. (1980), "Food poisoning from raw red kidney beans," *Brit Med J*, vol. 2, pp. 236-237.; A. Pusztai et al. (1981), "The toxicity of Phaseolus vulgaris lectins: Nitrogen balance and immunochemical studies," *J Sci Food Agric*, vol. 32, pp. 1037-1046.

19. http://www.westonaprice.org/soy-alert/689-ploy-of-soy.html, retrieved October 8, 2010.

Chapter 6

1. Ethan Waters, "DNA Is Not Destiny," *Discover* 27, no. 11, November 2006.

Chapter 8

1. Kaiser Permanente (July 8, 2008), "Keeping A Food Diary Doubles Diet Weight Loss, Study Suggests," *ScienceDaily*, retrieved August 17, 2010, from http://www.sciencedaily.com/releases/2008/07/080708080738.htm.

Chapter 11

1. Inspired by the Kurt G. Harris, MD, weblog post "There is No Such Thing as a Macronutrient, Part I—Fats," http://www.paleonu.com/panu-weblog/2011/1/29/there-is-no-such-thing-as-a-macronutrient-part-i-fats.html, retrieved March 2, 2011.

Chapter 12

1. *Diabetes Care,* 2009 Dec;32(12):2161-7. E-pub September 3, 2009.

2. Bennard, Imbeault, and Doucet, 2005, "Growth hormone, a major hormonal driver of lipolysis ('burning off your own body fat for energy') is raised after exercise.", M. J. Ormsbee et al., 2007, "Fat metabolism and acute resistance exercise in trained men," *Journal of Applied Physiology*, 102, 1767-72.

Resources

Visit—www.theonediet.com for weekly blogs, free downloads, success stories, recipes, and the latest information.

Follow us on Twitter—www.twitter.com/theonediet

Join us on Facebook—www.facebook.com/theonediet

The ONE Diet **Audiobook**—everything you need to know for those on the go; reinforce your own understanding, or a great gift for a busy friend. Available January 2012.

Change Directions—Georges Philips' companion book, especially for those planning positive life changes. Visit www.change-directions.com.

Authors' Web Sites

Georges Philips—www.georgesphilips.com
Simon Shawcross—www.simonshawcross.com

Other Web Sites of Interest

M. Doug McGuff, MD—www.bodybyscience.net
Kurt G. Harris, MD—www.archevore.com
Jimmy Moore—www.thelivinlowcarbshow.com
The International Network of Cholesterol Sceptics—www.thincs.org

Recommended Reading

Body by Science—Doug McGuff, MD, and John R. Little

Change Directions: Perceive It. Believe It. Achieve It.—
Georges Philips

Good Calories, Bad Calories/The Diet Delusion—Gary
Taubes

Influence: The Psychology of Persuasion—Robert Cialdini

My Little Book of Verbal Antidotes—Georges Philips and
Tony Jennings

Stop Thinking, Start Living: Discover Lifelong Happiness—
Richard Carlson

The Body By Science Question and Answer Book—Doug
McGuff, MD, and John R. Little

Notes

Notes

Notes

Notes

Notes

Notes

Lightning Source UK Ltd.
Milton Keynes UK
UKOW041935120313

207542UK00001B/17/P